AIDS, drugs and prevention

Perspectives on individual and community action

Edited by
Tim Rhodes and Richard Hartnoll

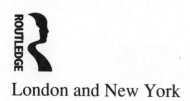

London and New York

First published 1996
by Routledge
11 New Fetter Lane, London EC4P 4EE

Simultaneously published in the USA and Canada
by Routledge
29 West 35th Street, New York, NY 10001

Routledge is an International Thomson Publishing company

Typeset in Times by
Ponting–Green Publishing Services, Chesham, Bucks
Printed and bound in Great Britain by
TJ Press (Padstow) Ltd, Padstow, Cornwall

British Library Cataloguing in Publication Data
A catalogue record for this book is available from the
British Library

Library of Congress Cataloguing in Publication Data
A catalogue record for this book has been requested

ISBN 0–415–10203–0 (hbk)
ISBN 0–415–10204–9 (pbk)

In memory of John K. Watters

Contents

Figures

Tables

Contributors

Marina Barnard is a Senior Research Fellow at the Centre for Drug Misuse Research, University of Glasgow. She has worked in the field of HIV/AIDS over the last seven years, conducting ethnographic work on drug injectors and their HIV risks. Her doctoral thesis was on gender differences in HIV risk behaviour. More recently she has looked specifically at female prostitutes' risks of HIV infection. She is co-author of two books with Neil McKeganey: *AIDS and Sexual Risk: Lives in the Balance* (Milton Keynes: Open University Press, 1992) and *Working on the Streets: Female Prostitutes and Their Clients* (Milton Keynes: Open University Press, 1996).

Robert Broadhead is a Professor in the Department of Sociology, University of Connecticut, Storrs, CT. He is the Principal Investigator of the Eastern Connecticut Health Outreach (ECHO) Project which is examining the dynamics of a peer-driven intervention. He is a graduate of the University of California, San Francisco, and his main areas of expertise include health sociology, the sociology of drugs and society and qualitative methodologies.

Richard Curtis is an ethnographer at National Development Research Institutes, Inc., New York. He is currently working on a project investigating HIV risk among youths in Brooklyn. His research interests include the structure of distributor and consumer groups in street-level drug markets, and law enforcement. He has recently completed a study of the impact of New York City's Tactical Narcotics Team on street-level drug markets in central Brooklyn.

Don C. Des Jarlais is Director of Research for the Chemical Dependency Institute of Beth Israel Medical Center, New York, Senior Research Fellow with National Development and Research Institutes, Inc., New York, and Professor of Community Medicine at Mount Sinai School of Medicine, New York.

Martin C. Donoghoe is currently with the Programme on Substance Abuse at the World Health Organisation (WHO), Geneva. He is involved in activities which aim to assess the extent, nature and social implications of drug use in countries worldwide. These include the development, field testing and promotion of epidemiological surveillance techniques and rapid assessment methodologies, particularly in developing countries. He is a co-author of the *WHO Multi-City Study on Drug Injecting and Risk of HIV Infection* (WHO/PSA, 1994) and has published widely on the HIV risk behaviour of injecting drug users.

Samuel R. Friedman is a Senior Principal Investigator with National Development and Research Institutes, Inc., New York, and has consulted for the United States National Institute on Drug Abuse and the WHO.

Jean-Paul C. Grund is the first Research Fellow in residence at the Lindesmith Center, a New York based drug policy and research institute, where he is engaged in developing harm reduction initiatives in former communist countries. He also has an appointment at the University of Connecticut on the Eastern Connecticut Health outreach (ECHO) Project. In the early 1980s he worked with the Dutch 'Junkiebonden', the first drug user self-organisations. He founded and directed Rotterdam's needle exchange.

Graham Hart is Assistant Director of the MRC Medical Sociology at the University of Glasgow and was previously a Senior Lecturer at University College London Medical School. He has researched and published widely in the areas of sexual and injecting risk behaviours for HIV infection. He is co-editor (with Peter Aggleton and Peter Davies) of the 'Social Aspects of AIDS' series. Recent titles include: *AIDS: Safety, Sexuality and Risk* (London: Taylor and Francis, 1995), *AIDS: Foundations for the Future* (London: Taylor and Francis, 1994) and *AIDS: Rights, Risk and Reason* (London, Falmer Press, 1992). He is also joint editor of the journal *AIDS Care* (Carfax Publishing).

Richard Hartnoll is the Principal Adminstrator responsible for coordinating European activities on the epidemiology of drug use at the European Monitoring Centre for Drugs and Drug Addiction, Lisbon. He previously worked at the Institut Municipal d'Investigacio Medica in Barcelona and at Birkbeck College, Unversity of London. His research interests include epidemiology, ethnography, evaluation of interventions, policy studies and multi-method approaches to studying drug use and drug use problems.

Douglas D. Heckathorn is a Professor in the Department of Sociology, University of Connecticut, Storrs, CT. He is the Co-Principal Investigator of the Eastern Connecticut Health Outreach (ECHO) Project and a former recipient of awards by the National Science Foundation. He is a graduate of the University of Kansas and his main areas of expertise include sociological theory, mathematical modelling and social organisation/collective behaviour.

Dagmar Hedrich is a psychologist working in the Pompidou Group Secretariat at the Council of Europe Headquarters in Strasbourg where she oversees the demand-reduction programme and the cooperation programme with central and eastern Europe on the epidemiology and prevention of drug use. Prior to this she worked as a researcher in a five-year follow-up of heroin users, and as the administrator in the drug policy department of the city of Frankfurt am Main.

Sheila Henderson has been a freelance researcher and consultant specialising in qualitative research and evaluation in the field of illicit drug use, young people and sexual health for four years. Prior to this she was based in the Research and Development Unit at the Institute of Drug Dependence, London. She has worked extensively for national and regional drugs agencies and information services, together with a range of relevant policy bodies in the major cities of England and Scotland. She has published widely on the subject of gender and drug use and is currently working on a book on young women's recreational drug use and sexuality.

Benny Jose is a Principal Research Associate at the Institute for AIDS Research, National Development and Research Institutes, Inc., New York. He is currently doing his doctoral dissertation on racial/ethnic aspects of AIDS among injecting drug users.

Stephen Koester is an Assistant Professor in the Department of Psychiatry at the University of Colorado Medical School and an adjunct Associate Professor of Anthropology at the University of Colorado, Denver. He is Co-Principal Investigator on two concurrent National Institute on Drug Abuse (NIDA) funded AIDS prevention research projects. His primary research interest in these projects has been on the context and mechanics of injection drug use. In addition to medical anthropology, he maintains a research interest in ecological anthropology. Recently, he completed a Fulbright Fellowship examining marine resource management issues in St Lucia, an island-nation in the Caribbean.

Neil McKeganey is Director of the Centre for Drug Misuse Research at the University of Glasgow. He has carried out a number of studies into various aspects of drug injectors' and female prostitutes' risk behaviour in relation to HIV. He is joint author with Marina Barnard of *AIDS, Drugs and Sexual Risk: Lives in the Balance* (Milton Keynes: Open University Press, 1992) and *Sex on the Streets: Prostitutes and Their Clients* (Milton Keynes: Open University Press, 1996).

Alan Neaigus is a Project Director at National Development and Research Institutes, Inc., New York on a project which examines HIV risk among young adults in a high-risk neighbourhood in Brooklyn. His current research interest is on the role of drug injectors' social networks in HIV risk and prevention. He is the author of a number of publications dealing with HIV risk and prevention among drug injectors and with evaluations of outreach interventions.

Cindy Patton is an Assistant Professor in the Department of English at Temple University, Philadelphia, Pennsylvania. She is author of several books on AIDS: *Sex and Germs: The Politics of AIDS* (Boston: South End Press, 1985), *Inventing AIDS* (New York: Routledge, 1990), *Last Served? Gendering the HIV Pandemic* (London: Taylor and Francis, 1994), and *Fatal Advice* (Durham, NC: Duke University Press, 1996).

Robert Power is Senior Lecturer in Medical Sociology at University College London Medical School. He was formerly Senior Research Fellow at the Centre for Research on Drugs and Health Behaviour, Charing Cross and Westminster Medical School, University of London. His main research interests lie in qualitative and action research, especially in relation to the development of community-based interventions. He has acted as a consultant for the WHO and United Nations Drug Control Programme in the practice and methodology of rapid assessment techniques. Recent publications include *Coping with Illicit Drug Use* (London: Tufnell Press, 1995).

Alan Quirk is a Researcher at the Centre for Research on Drugs and Health Behaviour, Charing Cross and Westminster Medical School, University of London. He is currently undertaking a qualitative study of risk, drug use and sexual safety among stimulant and opiate users and their sexual partners. His main research interests lie in qualitative studies of communication.

Tim Rhodes is Research Fellow at the Centre for Research on Drugs and Health Behaviour, Charing Cross and Westminster Medical School, University of London, where he is undertaking a number of qualitative studies into drug use, risk perception and sexual safety among drug users, people with the HIV infection and their sexual partners. His other research interests include medical sociology, qualitative methodology and the development and evaluation of community-based interventions. He is author of *Risk, Intervention and Change: HIV Prevention and Drug Use* (London: Health Education Authority, 1994), and is currently working on a book called *Risk and Behaviour: Sex, Drugs and Dangers in the Time of AIDS*.

Bruce Stepherson is the Director of the Center for AIDS Outreach and Prevention, National Development and Research Institutes, Inc., New York. He has worked extensively with Bronx–Harlem Needle Exchange since 1990 and is the first president of New York Harm Reduction Educators, Inc. He has written and presented on topics related to injecting drug use, IDU social networks, and issues which put IDUs at risk of HIV infection.

L. Synn Stern is a health educator who is currently completing an MPH at Hunter College in New York City. She helped establish needle exchange services in the Bronx, and the Eastern Connecticut Health Outreach (ECHO)

Project, and is a member of the health committee of Prostitutes of New York (PONY). She is working on a book on street survival in 'the Fourth World', safer self-injection and safer sex work.

Gerry V. Stimson is Director of the Centre for Research on Drugs and Health Behaviour, Charing Cross and Westminster Medical School, University of London and Professor of the Sociology of Health Behaviour at the University of London. He researches and writes on drug problems and drug policy, and has current interests in the sociology of public health and in public health interventions for drug users in developed and developing countries. He is co-editor (with John Strang) of *AIDS and Drug Misuse* (London: Routledge, 1990).

Meryl Sufian is an independent consultant in New York who has been conducting research and demonstration projects on drug use and HIV prevention. She is the author and co-author of several articles on HIV and ethnicity, HIV and risk reduction, and drug use. She received her Ph.D. from the City University of New York Graduate School.

John K. Watters was Associate Professor of Health Policy and Community Medicine at the University of California, San Francisco, and Director of the Urban Health Study. He was involved in the implementation and evaluation of AIDS prevention programmes in the United States from the mid-1980s up until his death. His research interests included the use of community-based approaches for increasing hepatitis B vaccinations among injecting drug users and the development of low-cost, high-adherence alternatives for anti-tuberculosis therapy among indigent inner-city populations.

Wayne Wiebel is an Associate Professor of Epidemiology at the University of Illinois at Chicago, School of Public Health. He is also Director of the Community Outreach Intervention Program at the School.

Acknowledgements

We are both indebted to the contributing authors who made this book possible. We would also like to express our thanks and gratitude to Monica Perez-Gomez and Jo Hooper for their help in preparing the final version of the manuscript. We also thank Heather Gibson and Fiona Bailey at Routledge for their editorial advice.

Tim Rhodes and Richard Hartnoll
London/Barcelona, 1995

Chapter 1

Individual and community action in HIV prevention

An introduction

Tim Rhodes

This book brings together a number of international contributions on the research, theory and practice of developing community-based HIV prevention interventions. This is achieved in three main ways. First, by examining the implications of research for understanding how and why individuals act as they do in response to the risk of HIV transmission; second, by discussing the implications of this research for developing health and HIV prevention interventions; and third, by exploring the aims and practice of innovative community-based HIV prevention among populations most affected by HIV and AIDS. The aim is to understand how individual actions are influenced by the social, cultural and political contexts in which such actions occur, and to explore how future HIV prevention interventions can target changes at the level of the individual as well as at the level of the community and wider social environment.

HEALTH PROMOTION AND BEHAVIOUR CHANGE

Recent developments in health promotion have advocated the need to balance individual and community action as a means of facilitating and enabling changes in individual and collective health status (Bunton and MacDonald, 1992). The 'new' public health movement of the 1980s promised to move beyond a biomedical understanding of individual health behaviour towards a new understanding which encompassed the social and environmental influences on individuals' health choices, perceptions and actions (Ashton and Seymour, 1990). It was recognised that not only should health interventions target individuals with the aim of encouraging individual behaviour changes, but, where necessary, interventions should also encourage changes in the communities and social environments of which these individuals were a part. In response, 'health promotion' became re-defined as the intersectoral activity which encourages possibilities for individual action as well as community action and changes in the social and political environment (World Health Organisational [WHO], 1986; Bunton and MacDonald, 1992).

Health promotion theory thus conceives of health as being a product not only of individual actions but also of actions which take place in the social contexts and environments in which individual behaviours occur. Individual actions, and individuals' desires or capabilities to change their behaviour, can be seen to be inextricably related to the 'social actions' of their communities, cultures or environments. The 'choices' individuals have and make about health, for example, are not simply a product of individual cognitive or rational decision-making. Rather, they are influenced by how other individuals think and behave and the social factors exogenous to individuals themselves which constrain or encourage the degree of 'choice' individuals can exercise.

The social factors which constrain or encourage individual choices and actions are many and varied. They may operate at the level of interpersonal interactions, as in the case of communication or 'negotiation' within sexual encounters where the actions or words of one individual have a direct bearing on the actions and words of the other. In behavioural situations where at least two individuals are present, choice of action is often a product of the *interaction* of individuals rather than something endogenous to individuals themselves. The social constraints on individual actions may also be community-oriented. An example of this is where group or community 'norms' influence what is considered to be appropriate, acceptable or 'normal' behaviour. Individual perceptions of social acceptability and 'normality' have a direct influence on how individuals behave. This is because individual actions which deviate from community norms are generally harder actions to make. Finally, the constraints on individual actions may also be politically oriented. An example of this is where local or state health and legal policies influence the degree to which individuals and communities can minimise their risks of health-related harm.

It is therefore an axiomatic principle of health promotion interventions that in order to encourage changes in the ways individuals think and behave it is often also necessary to encourage changes in the actions of their communities, cultures or environments. This is necessary so as to create the social conditions in which individuals are able – and can be encouraged – to exercise 'choice' about how they act in response to the risk of disease or illness. Health interventions are thus more likely to be effective if they encourage concomitant changes at the level of the individual, the community and the wider social and political environment.

HIV PREVENTION, RISK REDUCTION AND BEHAVIOUR CHANGE

Following the general principles of health promotion, the prevention of HIV infection requires an integrated approach to encouraging behaviour change which encompasses individual and social models of health intervention and change (Figure 1.1). Individual and social intervention approaches make different assumptions about the factors which influence risk and health

Intervention models	Intervention strategies	Assumptions about change	Nature of change
Individual approaches			
information giving	provision of information awareness raising	changes are required in individuals' knowledge and health beliefs	individual
individual empowerment	providing the means for individual change increasing self-efficacy increasing self-enablement	changes are required in individuals' self-efficacy to effect desired behaviour change	individual
Social approaches			
community action	peer education community participation community organisation social diffusion of change	changes are required in social norms and values about risk which influence individual health beliefs and behaviours	community
political action	political lobbying political activism policy change	changes are required in the social and political climate so that changes in social norms become possible	political

Figure 1.1 Individual and social approaches to HIV prevention

behaviour and how behaviour change is best achieved. Figure 1.1 illustrates how a comprehensive HIV prevention intervention strategy requires an integrated theoretical and methodological approach to encouraging individual, community and political action.

The HIV epidemic has brought new dimensions of risk. It has also brought about many changes. These changes have occurred in the everyday lives of the individuals and communities affected by HIV disease. They have also occurred in the ways health interventions aim to encourage risk reduction and behaviour change. The combination of medical uncertainty associated with the development of a vaccination against HIV and the public health urgency to prevent further HIV spread has encouraged the need for pragmatism in intervention responses which aim to prevent HIV transmission. This has facilitated what have come to be viewed as innovative styles of service delivery characterised by community-based interventions among populations most affected by HIV and AIDS.

For the most part, intervention responses have been based in a public health realism of the risks and dangers associated with an uncontrolled spread of HIV infection. The pragmatism which has characterised the emergence of HIV prevention responses in many countries has encouraged a recognition of the need to target changes in individual *and* community health. Yet while many HIV prevention interventions are 'community-based', they are rarely 'community-oriented'. Contemporary HIV prevention responses have been overwhelmingly focused on targeting individuals with the aim of encouraging individual behaviour change. In reality, few interventions have adopted methods which simultaneously aim to encourage changes in the social contexts or environments where individual actions take place. Even less often have interventions attempted to bring about changes in the policy or the political environment.

This leads to the question of how much practical impact the rhetoric of health promotion and the new public health has had. The language of HIV prevention gives much credence to the notions of 'enablement', 'empowerment' and the 'community'. Yet there are few HIV prevention interventions which systematically undertake 'community development' or which facilitate what can truly be seen to be 'community action' among members of affected communities themselves (Rhodes, 1994). The practice of most HIV prevention intervention falls short of the much-quoted ideals or principles of health promotion and the new public health movement (see WHO, 1986; Ashton and Seymour, 1990). The over-reliance on targeting individuals and individual behaviour changes alone restricts both the possibilities and parameters of change to individuals. What is needed are HIV prevention interventions that work *with* the community and not just *in* the community (Stimson *et al.*, 1994). This demands more than the *advocation* of an integrated approach to encouraging individual, community and political action. It also demands an *application* of these intervention methods in practice.

PERSPECTIVES ON INDIVIDUAL AND COMMUNITY ACTION

This book considers the diverse practices of individuals and interventions in the context of perspectives from research on individual and community action. The chapters which follow provide an overview of research on the social context of risk behaviour and health intervention among injecting drug users, female stimulant users, gay and bisexual men and female sex-workers. The focus of discussion is on the development of interventions oriented towards community action and community change. This book hopes to make advances in the theory, method and practice of community-oriented interventions among populations most affected by HIV and AIDS.

Individual action, HIV prevention and the policy environment

Most psycho-social models of health behaviour are individualistic in focus in that they seek to explain and predict the health behaviour of individuals by reference to their personal characteristics. These models, which emphasise the 'health beliefs' (Rosenstock, 1974), 'self-efficacy' (Bandura, 1977) and motivations and skills (Rosenstock et al., 1988) of individuals to behave in certain ways, tend to assume that individuals' decision-making on health choices is based on the perceived costs and benefits of action. Models of behaviour change that stem from these theories aim to enable individuals to have the knowledge and means to make healthy choices about their behaviour and lifestyles.

All of the chapters in this book share an appreciation of the limitations of individualistic models of health behaviour and behaviour change. They recognise that while providing pointers to individual behavioural intentions, they often fail to adequately capture the social dimensions or complexity of individual action. Chapter 2 (Gerry Stimson and Martin Donoghoe), for example, discusses the problems and possibilities associated with developing syringe exchange interventions. Such interventions aim to provide individuals with both the knowledge and the means to avoid HIV infection by injecting drugs safely. Yet, as Stimson and Donoghoe point out, despite the considerable success of syringe exchange interventions in the UK and Australian context, there are inherent limitations in these interventions by virtue of their individualistic focus. This restricts both the practical efficiency with which syringe exchange interventions can reach target populations and the effectiveness with which they can actually encourage individuals to change their injecting behaviour.

John Watters (Chapter 3) provides an additional perspective on how the social and political environment can influence the effectiveness of syringe exchange interventions. Whereas in the UK syringe exchange was adopted as part of a pragmatic public health response to prevent HIV and other blood-borne infections associated with injection, in San Francisco, as in many other states in America, the policy environment has impeded the development of such interventions. Watters traces the historical routes of resistance to syringe exchange in the United States, providing an incisive case-study of how the political environment can inhibit the development of what is seen, internationally, to be a pragmatic and effective method of HIV prevention. His chapter highlights the importance of community action in the absence of a 'healthy' policy environment and the necessity for political as well as individual and community change.

Richard Hartnoll and Dagmar Hedrich (Chapter 4) also examine the ways in which the local environment can influence the development of AIDS and drug policies and the implementation and impact of HIV prevention initiatives. Providing a case-study of the development of drug and intervention policies in Frankfurt, they explore how the aims and approach of HIV prevention interventions are influenced by tensions and dilemmas in the public and policy environment. Taken together, these three chapters aim to highlight how the nature of local and policy environments often have a direct bearing on whether and how interventions proceed. The effectiveness of HIV prevention not only depends on the theoretical or methodological approaches of specific interventions but also on whether the social conditions are conducive to action.

Community action and community change towards safer sex

There are two underlying reasons for developing community action interventions as a method of HIV prevention. The first concerns the inherent limitations of individually focused, one-to-one interventions in adequately reaching target populations within a specified community or social network. Community action interventions, in contrast, aim to encourage a system of peer support and participation which helps to overcome this problem. Second, as discussed in most of the chapters, interventions targeting individual behaviour changes alone are limited because they do not necessarily encourage the social conditions in which individuals can actually exercise 'choice'. The aim of community change interventions are thus to bring about changes in the community norms and practices which impede individual attempts at risk reduction, and reinforcements in the community norms and practices which endorse safer behaviour (Rhodes, 1993). These interventions encourage not only individual change but 'community change' – change which is oriented towards groups, networks or communities of individuals (Bracht, 1990).

Chapter 5 (Sheila Henderson), for example, draws on the implications of qualitative research among women who use 'dance' drugs for developing interventions which are oriented to the specific cultural mores of the 'rave' and 'club' scene. She argues that the recreational use of 'dance drugs' is inextricably bound up with the subcultural norms and values of the rave and dance club and that these subcultures provide their own channels of communication and influence for the social diffusion of intervention messages.

The effectiveness of social diffusion interventions oriented towards community change is discussed further by Graham Hart (Chapter 6). In a chapter reviewing both the rationale and evaluation of community-oriented HIV prevention interventions among gay and bisexual men in the UK and USA, he demonstrates, by way of specific intervention case-studies, that community action interventions can be effective in encouraging gay communities to endorse and sustain a 'norm' of safer sex. This chapter serves as a useful pointer to how community action interventions can facilitate the ease with which individuals make changes in their sexual risk behaviour.

In contrast to intervention studies among gay communities, there have been fewer attempts to examine the possibilities for peer education or community organising initiatives among female sex-workers. Drawing on their ethnographic research among female street-sex-workers in Glasgow, Scotland, Marina Barnard and Neil McKeganey (Chapter 7) examine some of the key obstacles and opportunities which exist for encouraging peer education interventions among women prostitutes. Their research highlights the importance of qualitative research in understanding the interplay of individual actions and social context. This has implications both for the ways in which future interventions among prostitutes prioritise the risks associated with HIV against other more immediate health risks and dangers, as well as for the ease with which interventions can encourage community change.

That community changes towards a 'norm' of safer sexual lifestyles can be encouraged and endorsed within some communities and not others, raises questions about the nature and diffusion of change within 'communities'. These points and their implications are among those discussed by Cindy Patton (Chapter 8). In her chapter outlining the key modes of activism and community organising which have evolved in response to HIV and AIDS, she explores the underlying tensions which exist between 'mainstream' and 'community' representations of 'safe sex'. Her discussion maps out how these struggles shed light on the ways in which knowledge and power are distributed in epidemic times and the implications of this for community and activist organising towards encouraging safer sexual practices. Her chapter points to the political dimensions of community work and the need for 'mainstream' preventive interventions to learn from the experiences and practices of affected communities themselves.

Peer education and community change among drug injectors

Chapters 9 to 14 examine the possibilities for community action and community change among drug injectors. Drawing on ethnographic and epidemiological research, these chapters highlight the limitations of research and intervention designs based on individualistic models of health behaviour.

On the basis of ethnographic observations undertaken among drug injectors in Denver, Colorado, Stephen Koester (Chapter 9) illustrates the value of anthropological and sociological research in describing the social dynamics and mechanics of injecting risk behaviour. His chapter, and Chapters 10 (Robert Power), 11 (Tim Rhodes and Alan Quirk) and 12 (Wayne Wiebel), show the practical value of ethnographic and sociological research in shaping intervention design and response.

These chapters share an appreciation of the need to understand the social context in which individual action takes place prior to developing community-oriented interventions to change drug use norms and practices. Robert Power (Chapter 10), for example, points to the importance of targeting drug using networks as a unit and agent of group mediated change. His chapter demonstrates the importance and utility of intervention strategies which encourage norm and group mediated change on drug use behaviours.

Interventions have had less success in encouraging drug users to change their sexual behaviour. In a chapter drawing on qualitative research on risk and sexual safety among heroin users in London, Tim Rhodes and Alan Quirk (Chapter 11) explore some of the key problems facing interventions which aim to encourage community change. They show first, how the everyday norms regulating drug using lifestyles encourage safer drug use practices yet unsafe sexual practices, and second, how the problem of sexual behaviour change brings to light some of the limitations in how effective peer education and community change interventions can be.

Building on ideas of how drug using networks can provide a focus for peer education, Wayne Wiebel (Chapter 12) gives practical examples of how ethnographic research can inform HIV prevention responses. This chapter provides an examination of a well-established model of subcultural change which aims to select, recruit and train 'indigenous leaders' within drug using networks as 'AIDS Prevention Advocates'. Jean-Paul Grund and colleagues (Chapter 13) also outline the theoretical and methodological foundations for a peer-driven intervention among drug injectors. This intervention model, located in East Connecticut, is based on a theory of group mediated social change which differs in approach to the Chicago model. Both chapters provide practical examples of how peer education methods can encourage changes in community as well as individual actions.

HIV prevention interventions among drug injectors may not only enlist drug users as peer educators but may also encourage community-wide mobilisation or organisation. Benny Jose and colleagues (Chapter 14) show how collective organising, as a method of community action and change, is distinct from peer education and social diffusion intervention. In their chapter, they describe the rationale, history and practice of collective organising among drug injectors in Brooklyn, New York. They provide evaluation data on the effectiveness of community organising initiatives in reducing sexual risk behaviour among drug injectors and their sexual partners. Taken together with Chapter 11, these data shed light on the possibilities for encouraging community changes in sexual norms among social networks of drug injectors.

Individual change requires social and political intervention

The chapters in this book illustrate how the relative success of HIV prevention interventions is inextricably linked to the social, cultural and political contexts in which they occur. At the outset, interventions require an understanding of the interplay of the individual and his or her context or environment. In the same way as individual 'choices' can be seen to operate within the constraints of group and community norms, collective action and change can be seen to operate within the constraints of the political and legal environment.

This book indicates that the challenge for all HIV prevention research and intervention is to recognise that there is often as much a need for community and political change as there is for individual behaviour change. This is because individual actions are influenced by 'social actions'. Whether these be the actions of communities or of policy makers, they often shape the extent to which individuals are in a position to exercise 'choice' about minimising risk and maximising safety. It is misleading to assume that by targeting individuals alone interventions will create the social conditions necessary for behaviour change. Future HIV prevention initiatives need to continue to encourage changes in the ways individuals behave but this also requires changes in the community and political environment.

REFERENCES

Ashton, J. and Seymour, H. (1990) *The New Public Health*, Milton Keynes: Open University Press.

Bandura, B. (1977) 'Self-efficacy: towards a unifying theory of behavioural change', *Psychological Review*, 84: 191–215.

Bracht, N. (ed.) (1990) *Health Promotion at the Community Level*, London: Sage.

Bunton, R. and MacDonald, G. (eds) (1992) *Health Promotion: Disciplines and Diversity*, London: Routledge.

Rhodes, T. (1993) 'Time for community change: what has outreach to offer?', *Addiction*, 88: 1317–1320.

Rhodes, T. (1994) *Risk, Intervention and Change: HIV Prevention and Drug Use*, London: Health Education Authority.

Rosenstock, I. M. (1974) 'Historical origins of the health belief model', *Health Education Monographs*, 2: 328–335.

Rosenstock, I. M., Strecher, V. J. and Becker, M. H. (1988) 'Social learning theory and the health belief model', *Health Education Quarterly*, 15: 175–183.

Stimson, G. V., Eaton, G., Rhodes, T. and Power, R. (1994) 'Potential development of community oriented HIV outreach among drug injectors in the UK', *Addiction*, 89: 1601–1611.

WHO (World Health Organization) and Canadian Public Health Association (1986) 'Ottawa Charter for Health Promotion', *Health Promotion*, 1: iii–v.

Chapter 2

Health promotion and the facilitation of individual change

The case of syringe distribution and exchange

Gerry V. Stimson and Martin C. Donoghoe

> Drug injectors can and will change their behaviour to reduce their own risk
> of HIV infection and, to a lesser extent, the risk of transmitting the virus
> to others.

That remarkable conclusion can be drawn from an accumulating body of
evidence from many countries. This evidence includes findings from evaluations of a wide variety of programmes that have been specifically designed
to promote and facilitate behaviour change among people who inject drugs;
from epidemiological and survey-based research of drug injectors in treatment, attending other helping agencies and in the community; and from
qualitative or ethnographic social and behavioural studies. A major public
health success story, which remains to be properly documented, will show
that from 1985 onwards innovative health promotion projects have brought
far-reaching changes in drug injectors' behaviour (Stimson, 1995; Des
Jarlais and Friedman, 1994). This is all the more extraordinary given that
before the HIV/AIDS era, many people working with drug injectors would
have been extremely pessimistic about the feasibility of encouraging such
changes. We now know that harm minimisation can achieve its objectives
and that health gains that fall short of abstinence from illicit and injecting
drug use can be achieved and can have a cumulative impact on the spread of
the HIV infection. The behaviour changes attained by drug injectors over-
shadow those in the general population. Drug injectors, in common with other
marginalised and stigmatised groups, have taken the lead in demonstrating
that people can respond to the threat of HIV infection.

RISK BEHAVIOUR AND HEALTH PROMOTION

A variety of innovative practices have been introduced to help prevent the
spread of HIV among drug injectors through syringe sharing and, to a far
lesser extent, from drug injectors to their injecting and non-injecting sexual
partners. Interventions to prevent transmission of HIV among drug injectors
have focused on drug use, drug injecting and syringe sharing. These include
interventions that seek to reduce syringe sharing, such as syringe distribution

and exchange, and those that encourage syringe hygiene, such as bleach distribution programmes. These interventions have, in the main, focused on encouraging changes in individuals' drug using and injecting behaviour, and less on their sexual risk behaviour. Whilst this focus on individual drug using, injecting and syringe sharing risk behaviour is a narrow one, it is eminently comprehensible in terms of the epidemiological dynamics of HIV infection. HIV is a behavioural disease, spread through intimate – and mainly shared – social activities, and its transmission is potentially under human control. Given that there is neither vaccination nor cure, prevention must focus in part on changing individual behaviours and encouraging personal responsibility. Public health, in the form of health promotion, has taken on board this challenge of enabling and facilitating behaviour change.

Most interventions designed to prevent HIV transmission have adopted a 'knowledge and means' approach to behaviour change. In its simplest form, this provides individuals with knowledge about risk and risk behaviour (e.g. the risk of HIV transmission through sharing syringes), along with providing them with the means to make changes in their risk behaviour (e.g. by providing them with sterile needles and syringes). As we will suggest later in this chapter, this approach was based on a new conception of the drug injector as a person concerned with and able to make rational decisions about their health. This essentially individualised notion of health behaviour is consonant with more generally held views about health promotion in the latter part of the twentieth century. In turn, we suggest that this provides a rather restrictive view of the nature of health behaviour, ignoring as it does the communal aspects of health and risk behaviour, and the social circumstances and social conditions which are often obstacles to behaviour change. To do this, we take syringe exchange as an example of an HIV prevention intervention based on a 'knowledge and means' model of behaviour change, and explore both the strengths and limitations of this approach.

THE HISTORY OF SYRINGE EXCHANGE: PROMOTING BEHAVIOUR CHANGE

Syringe exchange was a key aspect of innovative practices and interventions introduced to help prevent the spread of HIV among drug injectors. In many European countries, and in Australia and New Zealand, syringe distribution and exchange was a rapidly expanding area of work from the mid-1980s onwards. For many countries it was, and continues to be, of major significance in helping people who work with drug users to develop new aims, working practices, and working ideologies.

In Britain, the introduction of syringe exchange schemes heralded a major reorientation in the conceptualisation of the drug user and in the aims and practices of drugs services. The first syringe exchange schemes started in Britain in 1986. This was followed by a government-supported pilot experiment with fifteen schemes in 1987–88 (Donoghoe *et al.*, 1992). This pragmatic policy response was bold and controversial but deemed necessary because of rising levels of HIV infection, particularly in Edinburgh, Scotland. Syringe exchanges are now found in most towns and cities throughout England, Scotland and Wales. By the early 1990s there were over 250 syringe exchange sites in Britain and over thrity in London alone.

In the Netherlands, distribution and exchange programmes started slightly earlier than in Britain. In 1984, the first Dutch exchanges were established in Amsterdam in response to an outbreak of hepatitis B infection (HBV). Other Dutch cities implemented syringe exchange programmes and by 1990 there were approximately 130 exchange schemes in operation. In Sweden, despite laws limiting syringe availability, two schemes in the south of the country (Malmo and Lund) have had syringe exchanges since 1986. Distribution and/or exchange schemes are now found in many European countries.

In Australia the first exchange scheme was established on a trial basis in Darlinghurst, New South Wales (NSW) in November 1986. Needle and syringe exchange and distribution programmes then developed officially in all Australian states, although the number of sites and relative coverage varies from state to state. In NSW in 1992 there were thirty-two 'primary' exchanges and eighty 'secondary' outlets. This distinction (between outlets whose major purpose was to provide needles and syringes and those schemes operating from host agencies such as drug and alcohol treatment and community heath centres) is an interesting one paralleled by the distinction made in Britain between the relatively uncommon 'stand-alone schemes' and the proliferation of schemes established in existing agencies, for the most part in community-based drugs advice and information services. In NSW, in common with other Australian states, the most important exchange and distribution scheme, and certainly the most numerous in terms of sites, was the Pharmacy Guild Fitpack Scheme. This scheme enabled drug injectors to purchase from pharmacists specially designed packs of needles and syringes that double as safe disposal containers, with subsequent replacement packs provided free of charge. A variation on this system in Western Australia (WA), the SS5 Fitpack Project was established in 1987, and provided pharmacies with a pack of syringes to be sold to drug injectors at a cost of $3.00 (AUS). In 1990, 400 NSW pharmacies and 196 WA outlets were participating in Fitpack schemes. In Victoria a state-wide Needle-Syringe Exchange program (NSEP) was established in 1987. In 1990 Victoria had seventy-seven exchange outlets. In WA, the first syringe exchange scheme was established by a non-governmental organisation in 1987 and has operated from a number of sites since then. In common with other cities in Australia, Perth (WA) developed a mobile syringe exchange. Mobile exchanges were also common in other countries and seen as particularly useful in reaching drug injectors in rural areas where access to fixed site distribution points was difficult.

In the United States of America there was resistance to syringe exchange schemes and legal prohibition on the possession and distribution of syringes existed (and still exists) in many states (see Chapter 3). At the time when schemes were developing in Europe and Australia, most projects in the USA were clandestine and illegal: notable exceptions were those in New Haven, Portland, Boulder, Honolulu, Seattle and Tacoma. A privately run syringe exchange scheme was in operation in San Francisco from 1988 and, although it was the largest scheme in the United States, its legal status was unclear. Where legal schemes were permitted, they received no government funding and in the main operated outside of drug and treatment services.

Some schemes in Britain work in collaboration with retail pharmacies, and in Australia pharmacies work directly with both statutory and non-governmental HIV and drugs services. Outreach and mobile distribution and exchange operate in several countries including Australia, the Netherlands and Britain. Some exchanges in the United States have been little more than trestle tables on the sidewalk in high drug use areas. Some exchanges in Britain, and more commonly in Australia and the Netherlands, only provide exchange or distribution of syringes, and contact with drug injectors is kept to a minimum. Others have a variety of additional services and activities including the provision of primary medical care, drug and HIV counselling, sex counselling and access to HIV counselling and testing. Exchanges are variably linked to treatment and other help programmes and agencies. Sometimes, providing onward referral to treatment has been a condition of the scheme, as in an earlier ill-fated project in New York City which was conceived as 'a bridge to treatment'. Elsewhere the links to treatment programmes have been more tenuous. In Britain syringe exchanges often combine the distribution and disposal of syringes with access to drug counselling and treatment, and access to services not directly related to the provision of injecting equipment or drug related problems. Many schemes in Britain added primary medical and social care, including referral to other help and treatment agencies. It is not uncommon for schemes in Britain to provide help and advice with legal, financial and housing problems. This has not been the case in other countries, where wuch services for drug users are not provided or are provided as part of the general welfare system.

In Britain distribution of injecting equipment has been contingent, to some degree, on the return of used equipment. It was quickly learned, however, that insistence on a strict one-for-one exchange was impractical and most schemes operate within negotiable credit limits. Where other means of distribution have developed – for example pharmacy or shop sale and vending machines – the link with syringe disposal facilities and with drug counselling and other services may be more tenuous or non-existent. Some exchanges have deliberately maintained a policy of minimal contact in order to maximise participation by potential clients, but at a cost of missing opportuities for other intervention alongside needles and syringes.

EFFECTIVENESS OF INTERVENTIONS

There is considerable evidence that public health HIV prevention projects are successful. In Britain, the strategy to increase syringe distribution developed from observations that a shortage of syringes in Edinburgh, Scotland between 1981 and 1985 had contributed to high risk sharing behaviour and the rapid spread of HIV. Before the era of HIV/AIDS awareness (prior to 1986–87) the few studies that had looked at drug injecting indicated that between 60 and 90 per cent of drug injectors regularly shared needles and syringes. Studies since then have shown declining levels of syringe-sharing risk behaviour among many groups of drug injectors. In Britain, recent self-reported levels of syringe sharing have declined to less than 20 per cent. Those who continue to share do so with fewer people, and sharing is more discriminate (Stimson, 1995; Hunter et al., 1995). Ethnographic studies in Britain show that injectors no longer share as a matter of course and that syringe sharing is no longer part of the social etiquette of everyday drug use but an uncommon occurrence arising from exceptional circumstances (Burt and Stimson, 1993). These findings are similar to those from Rotterdam where syringe sharing is now disapproved of among drug injectors and 'not sharing' has become a social norm. These levels of risk behaviour are much lower than those still encountered in some parts of the United States (which are running at 60 to 70 per cent) and in other situations where there are limitations on the supply of syringes, such as in prisons.

Levels of HIV infection in most British cities have remained low in comparison to other countries, with a prevalence of less than 1 per cent, although HIV has been present among injectors in Britain since the early 1980s. The exceptions are Edinburgh and the north-east of Scotland (currently about 20 per cent), which faced the earliest outbreak of HIV infection, and in London where levels are in the region of 7 per cent (Stimson, 1995). In Edinburgh prevalence has declined and recent reconstructions of HIV incidence indicate a decline since a peak in the mid-1980s. Levels of infection in Britain have not reached those experienced by many other European and North American cities in the 1980s.

In Australia HIV prevalence rates remain low, in Sydney at under 5 per cent. In Amsterdam HIV infection rates among injecting drug users are about 30 per cent, but elsewhere in the Netherlands rates are less than 4 per cent. The rate for Amsterdam is relatively high when compared with Australian and most British cities, but seroconversion (incidence) rates have continued to decline and prevalence rates have stabilised. In Sweden HIV prevalence is lower among drug injectors in the south, where syringe exchanges were established in 1986 in Malmo and Lund, than elsewhere in the country where there are no syringe exchanges.

Most countries which adopted syringe distribution and other interventions that sought to minimise harm and reduce risk now have comparatively low or stabilised levels of HIV among injecting drug users. The high levels of HIV infection among drug injectors experienced in many other parts of the world, such as north-east India, Myanmar, Thailand and Brazil, have been avoided.

In summary, syringe exchanges have been established in many countries, they have reached many injectors (some coming into contact with a help service for the first time), they have enabled behavioural change and reduced risk, they have provided routes into treatment and have contributed other improvements in health and welfare. Cities and areas that provided syringe exchanges and other access to sterile injecting equipment early enough are characterised by low or medium but stable rates of HIV infection.

Despite these successes there are a number of limitations to syringe exchange programmes. These include selective and inadequate coverage of certain target populations. The international evidence shows that populations under-served include women, younger drug injectors, members of minority and other specific ethnic groups, those living in rural areas and injectors of drugs other than opiates. Schemes have not been successful in putting sexual behaviour change on the agenda, and an emphasis placed on changing syringe sharing may have been to the neglect of sexual risk. It is important to recognise that these limitations vary from city to city and country to country. However, our intention in this chapter is to address the fundamental assumptions of syringe distribution and exchange, and how these may lead to a limited perspective of what may be achieved and how it may be achieved. It is to this issue that we turn in the rest of this chapter.

MODELS OF SOCIAL BEHAVIOUR IN PUBLIC HEALTH

All social interventions, especially public health interventions, presuppose some general theory of social behaviour, which explains how and why the intervention is supposed to work. There will be an understanding – implicit or explicit – of the nature of social action, about the acquisition of knowledge, about the link between knowledge and behaviour, and about motivation to change behaviour.

Syringe exchange, in common with many other HIV preventive interventions, can be understood (retrospectively) in terms of a health belief model (Becker, 1984). This model presumes that when people are given knowledge about a disease or health problem they will perceive it as a threat, and will see the benefits of avoiding it. If they are also told how to avoid it, and given the means to do so, it is presumed that they will act to avoid it. In the case of syringe exchange, the idea (relatively poorly theorised at the time) was that drug injectors lacked knowledge about HIV and its transmission, and that they lacked the means to do anything substantial to avoid it. The syringe exchange programme combined a simple injunction based on knowledge about HIV transmission – 'don't share needles and syringes' – with the means for injectors to change their behaviour – the provision of sterile needles and syringes. A similar understanding underpinned the provision elsewhere of syringe decontaminants such as bleach. Given the legal constraints on syringe distribution in many parts of the United States, distribution of bleach provided drug injectors with the means to make the appropriate behavioural changes to avoid HIV infection should they share syringes.

There was considerable evidence to support the argument that a lack of means for sterile injection led to rapid spread of HIV infection. This was almost certainly the scenario in Edinburgh, and is still the case in many parts of the developing world where sterile equipment is in short supply or absent. In countries where the means to avoid infection have been available (as in Italy), the problem has been the lack of knowledge about the need to avoid HIV infection.

Hence the distribution of syringes was a practical, simple and cheap HIV prevention measure. It targeted the vehicle of the spread of the disease. It was also a 'democratic intervention', in that responsibility for avoiding infection and control over the means to do so were literally in the hands of the threatened population – the injectors who through the act of injection with previously used syringes placed themselves at risk of infection. Distribution of syringes was also relatively simple – even if in practice an expensive and complicated distribution system grew up around what could be a simple shopkeeping transaction. In suggesting that it was a democratic intervention, we are taking a cue from Illich's discussion of the social relations implicit in technologies (1973). Illich argues that technologies vary in the extent to which they are under the control of people who may benefit from them – those which are under the control of the beneficiary are more 'convivial' than those under the control of experts. The syringe is a simple technology – the user controls it and benefits from its use. It is useful to contrast the syringe with medical interventions that involve high levels of technology, or with psychological treatments that require high levels of training and competence of practitioners. In both of these cases, power is concentrated in the practitioner, in terms of access to and control over the means to change, and in terms of the specialist knowledge required to operate the equipment or undertake the therapy. Syringe distribution also gained popularity among many drugs workers and social activists because it was consonant with freedom-of-choice arguments proposed by populist-minded social workers with their desire to 'empower' and 'enable' clients. It is also worth noting that syringe distribution is not inconsistent with right-wing ideas about rolling back the frontiers of the state and making populations responsible for choices about their destiny.

RETHINKING THE DRUG USER

But syringe distribution in itself would not work unless the target population were amenable to, or could be persuaded to adopt, the intervention. A public health strategy based on a health belief model would not be successful unless the target population were particularly receptive to it. Many externally led social interventions fail because of the targeted social group's inability to comprehend or accept the rational model of behaviour that the intervention presumes.

With syringe exchange programmes the technology itself (the sterile disposable hypodermic syringe) was already part of the drug injectors' repertoire (though this may not be the case in developing countries where makeshift home-made injection equipment is used). The requisite change was that injectors would make efforts to obtain and use sterile needles, in preference to sharing old ones with others. This assumes that drug injectors are interested in their health, and enthusiastic about avoiding disease. This was not an image of the drug injector that would have been countenanced by many people working in the field in the mid-1980s, nor indeed is it an image of the drug user that would be understood or accepted in many parts of the world today.

Public health interventions therefore include conceptions of the *particular* characteristics of the target group – in other words, what sort of people they are, and why they might find the intervention acceptable. The 'interventionist gaze' includes ideas about the psychology of the target group, their concerns and values, and their relationships with others. These characteristics are in part descriptive. But they are also used proactively: they are an essential element of the ideological work that 'product champions' use to try to convince policy-makers that intervention is necessary, and to convince the target audience that they need the proffered service. This helps encourage changes in public views of the group and in the target population's conception of itself.

Thus in addition to an implicit 'knowledge and means' strategy, there is an accompanying vision of the nature of the drug users and the nature of drug use. These ideas may not have been clearly formulated at the time, except by public health polemicists – as is often the case, theorising about interventions often comes after their adoption. Rather, the ideas are part of the assumptive logic of proposing and pursuing the new strategy. We have to turn to various and scattered sources to tease out the underlying discourse on the nature of the drug injector that developed in the late 1980s.

AIDS did indeed prompt a major reconceptualisation of the drug injector, as has been discussed elsewhere (Stimson, 1989, 1994, 1995; Stimson and Lart, 1991, 1994). First, the reconceptualisation emphasised choice in social behaviour. It assumed, and hoped, that drug users were capable of making inherently rational decisions about their health. Previous characterisations of the drug user have often emphasised their sociopathology, or their psychopathology (as in psychiatric and psychological theories that view addiction, dependence or intoxication as interfering with freedom of choice and rational action). In contrast, the new view of the injector helped to *depathologise* drug use, and encourage a view of drug injectors as responsible for their actions. This was a humanising view. The proposition that 'drug users are people' was reflected in the shift in terminology, away from primary statuses such as 'addict' or 'intravenous drug abuser' to behavioural descriptions such as 'people who inject drugs'.

Second, the reconceptualisation assumed that drug users were concerned about their health. The 'health-conscious drug user' was considered to be responsive to public health and educational information, able to engage in rational health planning, and to balance long-term threats against short-term pleasures (Stimson, 1989). This view supposed that drug users share with others an inherent rationality when it comes to health – that they and the rest of the population share the same 'health values'. This had the advantage in terms of HIV prevention in that in theory it counters the marginalisation of injectors. This new image was in distinct contrast to previous character-isations of the drug addict that focused on such cultural roles as the 'bohemian', 'hedonist', 'outlaw' and 'rebel', or viewed the addict as the occupant of a self-chosen and self-destructive sick role. This last role, with the indulgence in sick appearance and dependence on drugs (and, in the case of male addicts, supportive females) resonated with strong cultural ideas linking sickness with creativity, self-awareness and sensitivity as has been discussed by Susan Sontag with reference to tuberculosis (Sontag, 1977), and by Alethea Hayter (1968) with reference to the Romantic poets and their use of opium. Interestingly, the logic of this new view might be to devalue the special characteristics that would be claimed by some drug users – to promote what could be called a *de-culturisation* of the drug user. It sought to normalise drug use, and to show that drug injectors are just like anyone else, except they have chosen to inject drugs; rather than viewing them as less deserving than others, the implication is that like other citizens they have rights to health care, to travel, to bear children, and – perhaps – to use drugs.

Third, the reconceptualisation means that addiction to drugs *per se* was no longer a target for interventions. The focus was on the specific risk behaviours: drug use itself may not now be viewed as problematic behaviour, except in so far as it may be associated with harmful outcomes to health. Addiction came to have less relevance than the act of injecting, and furthermore, injecting itself could pose hazards to health even in the absence of dependence. Abstinence from drugs was therefore no longer the main target for drugs workers and others engaged in HIV prevention activities. Instead, workers came to focus on particular aspects of risks associated with drug use. Now targeted were the small changes in health behaviour which were seen as having a major impact on individual and public health through the prevention of transmission of the HIV infection. Physical health was now on the agenda. Before the era of AIDS, drugs workers had not been especially interested in health *per se*: their interest was in working with drug users' minds.[1] In an AIDS era, ideas of harm minimisation and safer drug use dominated: in turn there was a transfer of these ideas to other areas of health risk including hepatitis B and C and tuberculosis, and in providing primary health care, and health promotion advice (about nutrition, exercise, sleep and so on).

Finally, the new view of drug users entailed a redefinition of their relationships with others. The occupational language for drugs workers now included words such as 'enabling' and 'empowering' clients; making services 'accessible', and making them 'user friendly'. This was a change from professional dominance (Freidson, 1975) to more egalitarian interactions. The credibility of the doctor was supported by symbols of distance and difference from patients: the credibility of the drugs worker was displayed by the adoption of symbols of closeness and similarity. The suit (a symbol of office-based activity [Berger, 1980]) and the office were swapped for the dress of the street. 'Street credibility' took over from professional credentials.

THE INDIVIDUALISATION OF PUBLIC HEALTH THROUGH HEALTH PROMOTION

All this seemed very new, and special, to the field of drugs. But how special was it? In the latter part of the twentieth century the emphasis in public health in general had already shifted to the individual body and to choice of lifestyle. Public health became equated with the promotion of healthier ways of living. Brian Turner epitomised this in his caricature of the 'monogamous jogger' – the health-conscious citizen aware of his or her responsibility to the state for being healthy (Turner, 1984). Thus, the locus for good health came to be placed in the hearts, minds, mouths and muscles of individual citizens. This model of public health was very different from models of public health in earlier periods, when improvement in the health of the nation through public health activity was seen to result from collective measures to influence an environment over which individuals had little influence. The focus then was on such matters as housing, working conditions, sanitation, the water supply, and the quality of food products. Later, the public health effort shifted to protecting populations from infectious diseases which could not be controlled by the individual – one thinks of mass immunisation campaigns. In the last quarter of the twentieth century the emphasis for health promotion has shifted to a focus on changes in the way individuals behave. The syringe exchange strategy was thus constrained within a late-twentieth-century model of individualism and health. Some of the elements of this have been discussed elsewhere (Stimson and Lart, 1991). The vehicle for this is services delivered in and from agencies by professional workers to individual clients.

There is a certain irony that when professionals talk of 'enabling' or 'empowering' their clients, they are encouraging them to be more sophisticated consumers of services provided by professionals. Indeed the term 'client', at first sight seemingly more benign that the term 'patient', does not break free from the implication of a dependent relationship on a professional worker. The individualism that characterised the therapy of the drug clinic was now mirrored in the provision of individual advice and counselling on risk behaviour.

This is not to deny the enormous feats that syringe distribution and other similar HIV preventions have achieved, both in enabling behaviour change and in facilitating a more egalitarian and humanitarian vision of working with drug users. Syringe distribution remains a key element, and one that is urgently needed in many countries. The point rather is that the limitations of the approach are not just operational, but also in the overall vision.

In the dominant health promotion model that was found in syringe exchange, 'sharing' of syringes was thought of almost entirely as a matter of individual volition. However, in our view, the health choices that people make, and the behaviours they choose to pursue, are not independent of the context in which those choices are made and that behaviour occurs. The HIV prevention field has focused on syringe 'sharing', and at the same time has ignored the essentially social nature of 'sharing' as a behaviour involving two or more people. Sharing takes place in a particular social context, and in the context of the resources that those people have for being in a position to make healthy choices about their lives. Facilitating behaviour change therefore necessitates more than the counselling of individuals to change their behaviour. It requires encouraging and facilitating changes in communities or populations of drug injectors. This calls for actions that will lead to changes in the norms and practices of drug using groups, so that 'not sharing' becomes the norm, and so that HIV protective behaviours become mutually reinforced and reciprocated. In practical terms, this means that people who use syringe exchanges and other services should be more involved in promoting change in the beliefs and behaviours in the drug using community (Rhodes, 1993). Ultimately, the objective is to bring about changes in the everyday social etiquette of drug use (Burt and Stimson, 1993), so that measures to avoid the transmission of HIV infection are implemented and sustained as part of the daily routine of drug users. As has been suggested elsewhere, the strategy has to make use of the fact that 'the social networks through which HIV is transmitted are the same social networks that may be co-opted for HIV prevention' (Stimson *et al.*, 1994).

Thus far many (but not all) public health activities to prevent the spread of HIV infection have had little concern with the dynamics of populations, and little understanding of the ways in which behaviours occur within communities. To move beyond the current limitations will necessitate re-thinking the role that public health interventions such as syringe distribution and exchange may play in transforming everyday patterns of drug use.

NOTE

1 We are grateful to Rachel Lart for this interpretation.

REFERENCES

Becker, H.S. (ed.) (1984) *The Health Belief Model and Personal Health Behaviour*, Thorofare, NJ: Charles B. Slack.

Berger, J. (1980) 'The Suit and the Photograph', in *About Looking*, pp. 26–27, London: Writers and Readers Publishing Cooperative.

Burt, J. and Stimson, G.V. (1993) *Drug Injectors and HIV Risk Reduction: Strategies for Protection*, London: Health Education Authority.

Des Jarlais, DC and Friedman, S.R. (1994) 'AIDS and the use of injected drugs', *Scientific American*, February: 56–62.

Donoghoe, M.C., Dolan, K.A. and Stimson, G.V. (1992) *Syringe Exchange in England: An Overview*, London: Tufnell Press.

Freidson, E. (1975) *Profession of Medicine: A Study of the Sociology of Applied Knowledge*, New York: Dodd, Mead.

Hayter, A. (1968) *Opium and the Romantic Imagination*, London: Faber & Faber.

Hunter, G. M., Donoghoe, M.C., Stimson, G.V., Rhodes, T. and Charmers, C. P. (1995) 'Changes in the injecting risk behaviour of injecting drug users in London: 1990–1993', *AIDS*, 9: 493–501.

Illich, I.D. (1973) *Tools for Conviviality*, London: Calder & Boyars.

Rhodes, T. (1993) 'Time for community change: what has outreach to offer?', *Addiction*, 88: 1317–1320.

Sontag, S. (1977) *Illness as Metaphor*, Harmondsworth: Penguin Books.

Stimson, G.V. (1989) 'AIDS and HIV: the challenge for British drug services' (Fourth James Okey Lecture), *British Journal of Addiction*, 85 (3): 329–339.

Stimson, G.V. (1994) 'Minimising harm from drug use', in J. Strang and M. Gossop (eds) *Responding to Drug Misuse: The British System*, Oxford: Oxford University Press.

Stimson, G.V. (1995) 'AIDS and drug injecting in the United Kingdom 1987 to 1993: the policy response and the prevention of the epidemic', *Social Science and Medicine*, 41(5): 699–716.

Stimson, G.V. and Lart, R. (1991) 'HIV, drugs and public health in England: new words, old tunes', *International Journal of the Addictions*, 26 (12): 1263–1277.

Stimson, G.V. and Lart, R. (1994) 'The relationship between the state and local practice in the development of national policy on drugs', in J. Strang and M. Gossop (eds) *Responding to Drug Misuse: The British System*, Oxford: Oxford University Press.

Stimson, G.V., Eaton, G., Rhodes, T. and Power, R. (1994) 'Potential development of community oriented HIV outreach among drug injectors in the UK', *Addiction*, 89: 1601–1611.

Turner, B. (1984) *The Body and Society: Explorations in Social Theory*, Oxford: Basil Blackwell.

Chapter 3

Americans and syringe exchange

Roots of resistance

John K. Watters

No modern public health issue has aroused more political ardour, fear, and public imagination than AIDS. The emergence of the AIDS epidemic has significantly changed clinical and biomedical research priorities on a global scale. The growing numbers of injection drug users (IDUs) caught in the epidemic has focused additional attention on both the drug users and the health and social policies which affect them. In the United States, injection drug use accounted for 25 per cent of the 401,749 AIDS cases diagnosed up to June, 1994, and was the second largest risk category for AIDS, following gay/bisexual males (US Centers for Disease Control and Prevention, 1994). An additional 4 per cent were reported as cases involving heterosexual contact with known IDUs. Gay and bisexual men with drug injection histories accounted for another 6 per cent of AIDS cases. Just under 1 per cent of AIDS cases were classified as paediatric exposure due to injection drug use or sex with an IDU. Thus, at least 36 per cent of AIDS cases diagnosed in the United States through June 1994 were associated with injection drug use. This estimate is conservative, as there are another 35,103 adult and paediatric cases that are of unknown relation to injection drug use or IDUs. Nevertheless, the heightened attention health care policy and research have received as a result have had little impact on the direction or content of substance abuse policy in the United States.

Nowhere are the reasons for this intransigence in substance abuse policy better illustrated than in the ongoing debate surrounding the acceptability of syringe exchange as a prevention measure to slow the spread of HIV among IDUs. Many other industrialised countries have chosen to include increased access to sterile injection equipment, including needle exchange programmes, in their AIDS prevention portfolios, including Australia, Canada, Great Britain, Holland, and Sweden (see Chapter 2). Yet with a handful of exceptions, health policy in the United States remains locked in a protracted debate over the safety, efficacy, and morality of syringe exchange. What is it about America and the American mind that have so constrained public health policy with respect to confronting the HIV epidemic among IDUs? Why are disease prevention objectives held secondary to illusive drug abuse prevention and law enforcement objectives?

Opponents of legal access to syringes for drug users base their opposition on two assumptions. First, that measures such as syringe exchange programmes have not been conclusively proven to reduce new HIV infections in controlled studies. Second, opponents have argued that any loosening of restrictions on access to drug paraphernalia will undermine drug abuse prevention efforts by sending a mixed message which condemns drug use on the one hand, but condones it on the other by supplying the tools necessary for injecting. Some have argued that if AIDS is a possible outcome of drug abuse, then drug users should be held accountable for their decision to inject drugs, even if this means infection with an incurable disease. On the other hand, numerous studies in Europe and North America have concluded that syringe exchange programmes are unlikely to do much (if any) real harm in terms of stimulating additional injection drug use and appear to play a significant role in reducing needle-related HIV transmission risks (Lurie *et al.*, 1993). Proponents of syringe exchange programmes have argued that they are an important means to engage drug users in the public health system, provide education, and make referrals to much-needed health and social services (including drug treatment) where available (Hartgers *et al.*, 1989; van den Hoek *et al.*, 1989; Purchase *et al.*, 1989). There is growing evidence that access to clean injection equipment and syringe exchange are associated with lower rates of infectious disease (Nelson *et al.*, 1991; Kaplan and Heimer, 1992; Friedman, S. R. *et al.*, 1994) and less risky behaviour among drug injectors (Buzolic, 1988; Des Jarlais *et al.*, 1989; Hart *et al.*, 1989; Ljunberg *et al.*, 1991; Lurie *et al.*, 1993; Pye *et al.*, 1989; Stimson, 1989; Watters *et al.*, 1994). Consequently, syringe exchange programmes are likely to help reduce the risks of new HIV infections in this group, their sexual partners, and their offspring. At the same time there is no published evidence that these programmes have had any impact on stimulating drug abuse. To understand American resistance to syringe exchange, it is necessary to consider the historical and ideological context in which this opposition has developed. This chapter seeks to identify the principal roots of American resistance to syringe exchange.

EARLY AMERICAN RELIGIOUS THEMES: PURITAN DOCTRINE AS METAPHOR

While the United States is a culturally diverse society, in many respects the dominant culture reflected in its traditions and norms is derived from the early New England colonies. The early colonies were founded by expatriated religious zealots, and the religion was Calvinism. The Puritans who took up residence in the New England colonies were religious pilgrims who had rejected the ceremony and pomp of the Church of England and supplanted it with a strong and rigid set of moralistic beliefs. The First Great Awakening (1740–41) was a period of spiritual rebirth in which many enduring American institutions have their origins. Among these are the roots of the American tradition of missionary work; the foundations of the slave abolition movement; and the creation of a number of America's first colleges and universities. Jonathan Edwards (1703–58) emerged as a leading Puritan minister and intellectual in New England. His writings and charismatic style made him one of the principal religious leaders of his time. He is credited both with having launched the 'revival of 1734' and with playing a major role in the Great Awakening (Smith, 1992). Edwards preached a fiery end to sinners. His eloquent enumerations of the eternal horrors of hell served as the model for much of what later came to be aped from the pulpits, wagons, and tents of Pentecostal and evangelical preachers over the ensuing 250 years. In his sermon 'Sinners in the Hands of an Angry God', delivered at Enfield, Connecticut on 8 June 1741, Edwards portrayed the consequences that await the unregenerate soul and coined the rhetoric for holy-rollers and hellfire-spouting preachers to follow. Sinners, he wrote:

> are as great heaps of light chaff before the whirlwind; or large quantities of dry stubble before devouring flames . . . The *devil* stands ready to fall upon them, and seize them as his own . . . There are in souls of wicked men those hellish *principles* reigning, that would presently kindle and flame out into hell fire, if it were not for God's restraints . . . [Sinners] are held in the hand of God, over the pit of hell; they have deserved the fiery pit, and are already sentenced to it; and God is dreadfully provoked, his anger is great toward those that are actually suffering the executions of the fierceness of his wrath in hell . . . the devil is waiting for them, hell is gaping for them, the flames gather and flash about them, and would . . . swallow them up . . . They have no refuge, nothing to take hold of; all that preserves them from moment to moment is the mere arbitrary will, and uncovenanted, unobliged forbearance of an incensed God.
>
> (Edwards, 1741)

For Edwards and his Puritan followers, sinners were relegated to a pitiless eternity of torment. This Puritan vision of harsh punishment of unredeemed sin can be viewed as the metaphor for the treatment of drug users in twentieth-century America and continues to drive public policy governing the use of psychoactive substances. This metaphor relegates moral profligates to the most excruciating consequences for their wilful departures from piety.[1] And so it is with drug users. Certainly, America is not alone in its heritage of punishment of religious heretics. Few cultures are. Yet somehow, unlike the leaders of the European Inquisitions, the early Puritans retained the status of cultural heroes to a surprisingly large segment of American society. In this environment, underlying moralistic themes continue to re-emerge. Across a broad spectrum of political and religious thought, early Puritan themes continue to serve as boundaries which define what Americans should be in terms of what they should not become. Many Americans seek a 'moral compass' in times of rapidly changing social conditions. The *neo-Puritans* seek to re-apply the moral and theological template left by Calvinist theologians, such as Jonathan Edwards, to contemporary society. Threatened by a departure from the familiar, traditional values of America's pre-industrial, agrarian past, the rhetoric and imagery of Edwards and other Great Awakening theologians provides a metaphor for interpreting changes in American society. For such individuals, AIDS is viewed as the will of an outraged God which is visited upon those sinners who have engaged in drug abuse or in forbidden and sinful sexual acts.

In the United States, neo-Puritanism has developed into a major political movement. Led by charismatic missionaries, a latter-day 'moral crusade' is being waged using the vehicles of mass-marketing, television, lobbying, and power politics. The putative object of this contemporary mission is the transformation of secular America into the pious, Christian enclave en-visioned by Jonathan Edwards 250 years ago. Perhaps the best known and most powerful of the television evangelists is the Revd Jerry Falwell. Falwell founded and led the 'Moral Majority', a well-known Christian fundamentalist organisation of more than 500,000 members. The religious doctrine espoused by Falwell is derived largely from early American Puritans. Falwell waged a pragmatic campaign to influence American policy on such issues as abortion, homosexuality, pornography, defence spending, sanctions for South Africa, and aid to the Contras. Like other Christian fundamentalists, Falwell views AIDS as divine and wilful intervention on the part of an incensed God. Communities such as San Francisco, New York, and Los Angeles, and other venues popular among gays because of acceptance of gay lifestyles, are seen as the literal equivalents of Sodom and Gomorrah. Falwell has stated that 'AIDS is a lethal judgement of God on ... sin ... and it [AIDS] is the judgement of God on America' (Lattin, 1988).

Falwell's is an apocalyptic view of the public health crisis. And it is in his use of the considerable political might of his organisation and its sympathisers that we see articulated one of the principal ideological and theocratic roots of resistance to syringe exchange. Beyond the biblical imagery and skilful use of early Calvinist themes is an impressive political machine capable of exerting massive pressure on elected officials and political bureaucracies. An example of this political sophistication and power can be seen in events leading to the successful veto of the 1988 Civil Rights Bill. The bill, approved by Congress, strengthened anti-discrimination laws and would have prohibited discrimination in hiring and firing based on sexual preferences. Falwell distributed a letter to members of the Moral Majority, describing the bill as 'the greatest threat to religious freedom and traditional values ever passed'. The outpouring of calls to Congress intended to discourage the anticipated override vote was prodigious. Over 80,000 calls per hour were made to members of the Senate by Falwell's followers, effectively discouraging the anticipated override vote (Lattin, 1988). Faced by an overwhelming barrage of objection, the two-thirds override vote failed, and the veto held. Not only did Falwell achieve his immediate political objective of defeating the bill, but he demonstrated the potency of his political strategy and backing. For most of the 1980s, religious extremists (and fear of their wrath) determined the content of the American response to AIDS (Francis, 1992) down to the details of language and graphics in prevention brochures and pamphlets. Consequently, the religious right has played a pivotal role in the development of health policy relative to AIDS in the United States.

Parallel to Edwards' rhetoric, liberalisation of drug and anti-paraphernalia laws is viewed by neo-Puritans as heresy. Those who have argued for decriminalisation of drugs claim that adult citizens in a free society have the moral freedom, or *right*, to make decisions regarding their own intake of recreational substances (Husak, 1992). The opposing view has frequently been placed on a moral foundation: that the individual has a moral *obligation* to moderate his or her behaviour by avoiding drugs. It is useful to remember that the abhorrence of drug and alcohol use is such a powerful theme in American social history that earlier in this century the United States Constitution was actually amended to prohibit recreational use of alcohol.

Just as military heroes have emerged from the tumult of armed conflict, so too have numerous political careers been defined in the service of the suppression of drugs and those who use them. American 'pharmaphobia' is so deeply ingrained that no serious American politician or political bureaucrat can really question the assumptions that undergird it. In mid-December 1993, the Surgeon-General of the United States, Dr Joycelyn Elders, touched off a firestorm of controversy by suggesting that decriminalisation of illicit drug use be systematically studied, and that marijuana be evaluated by the US Food and Drug Administration as a possible treatment for glaucoma and iatrogenic nausea. Dr Elders' comments proved embarrassing to the Clinton Administration, which moved quickly to underscore President Clinton's opposition to the concept. While Dr Elders simply suggested the matter be objectively studied, the response from critics and the White House illustrates how those who question America's virulent anti-drug doctrine are viewed as heretics. Dr Elders, stunned by the strength of reaction to her comments, later remarked that 'the level of personal attack was a shock'. Dr Elders quickly learned through this punishing episode that merely suggesting an evaluation of criminal sanctions against drug use in contemporary American society is tantamount to questioning the existence of the devil in eighteenth-century America. It is within this ideological nexus that attempts at harm reduction – including syringe exchange – must be placed. Consequently, one of the principal roots of resistance to syringe exchange can be found in the overall religious and theological history and current climate of American thought involving the non-medical use of drugs.

AMERICAN NARCOTICS CONTROL POLICY: SIN, MEDICINE AND THE LEGISLATION OF MORALITY

Over the past 120 years laws have been enacted to regulate access to drugs and the means of their delivery (Musto, 1973). These include prescription laws, regulation of hypodermic equipment in all but ten of the fifty states, and drug paraphernalia laws that prohibit pipes, syringes, and other tools and materials used to ingest drugs. As of this writing (Autumn 1994), forty-five state jurisdictions in the United States have steadfastly retained drug para-phernalia laws that prohibit possession of hypodermic syringes for non-medical use. In all but ten states (which also have syringe prescription laws), these anti-paraphernalia laws are the principal mechanism used for the suppression of syringe exchange programmes that have been implemented by volunteer health workers. Despite the resilience of these laws, they are relatively recent, many having been enacted in the 1970s and 1980s.

At the beginning of the nineteenth century, American drug policy was more *laissez-faire*. There were no federal laws regulating possession or sale of heroin, morphine, cocaine, or marijuana. The key impetus for the criminal-isation of drug use over the ensuing years was the characterisation of drug users as moral reprobates: seducers who facilitated the descent of the innocent into a welter of sin and degradation (Epstein, 1977). Reminiscent of Edwards' imagery of the unregenerate soul, xenophobic white Americans fell easy prey to lurid tales of drug use among the 'criminal classes' and non-whites during the late-nineteenth and throughout the twentieth centuries. For example, the small amount of cocaine used as an ingredient in cola drinks (*circa* 1900) was reported to incite black men to rape white women. Opium smoking by the Chinese was also attributed to moral corruption (of white women). These reports were used to justify a rash of state-level initiatives that sought to control access to certain drugs (Musto, 1973).

In the latter half of the nineteenth century, various states began to enact prohibitions against drug use. Not until the early twentieth century did the United States government enter the fray by enacting two federal laws directed at bringing narcotics traffic under federal control. These were the 1911 Opium Exclusion Act, and the 1914 Harrison Act. The Opium Exclusion Act was stimulated by concern that Chinese nationals, involved in the opium trade, were using the drug to seduce white women. The Harrison Act, essentially a tax law, served as the basis for the United States government to regulate (by abolition) a growing clinical enterprise involving cocaine and morphine 'maintenance' practices conducted by physicians. Heroin maintenance clinics, initiated both before and after the turn of the century, were facilities where addicts could receive heroin and/or morphine from physicians. Addic-tion maintenance clinics were closed across America in the decade following the 1914 passage of the Harrison Anti-narcotics Law. In the federal attack on the heroin maintenance clinics, the same moral revulsion formerly reserved for the addict was vented on the physicians who were seen to pander to the morally reprehensible practice of taking narcotics. By 1922, several thousand American physicians had been arrested under the vague powers enfranchised by the Harrison Law. Addiction maintenance would remain illegal in the United States until the late 1960s when Drs Vincent Dole and Mary Nyswander published a series of articles on the utility of the synthetic narcotic agonist, methadone hydrochloride, as a substitute maintenance drug in the treatment of heroin addicts (Dole and Nyswander, 1965, 1967; Dole *et al.*, 1968). The pioneering work of Dole and Nyswander was translated into a public drug treatment system during the early 1970s under the Republican Administration of Richard M. Nixon as a cornerstone in an anti-crime domestic policy, thereby ushering in the modern era of methadone treatment.

A second major impact of the Dole and Nyswander efforts was the *medicalisation* of drug abuse treatment. By having a 'medicine' that could be offered in the context of 'treatment', the physician was re-introduced to the medical practice of addiction maintenance for the first time since the 1914 Harrison Law. While still not the highest status speciality for physicians, addiction treatment with methadone has become a significant if not principal mode for the medical treatment of addicts in the United States. Through such treatment, IDUs may achieve some degree of release from the economic and logistical burdens of continued, multiple, daily injections of heroin. As persons with a bona fide, diagnosed medical condition who are receiving medical treatment, society can view and treat them differently from IDUs who do not elect to struggle against their chemical dependencies. Since faith in science and medicine have replaced much of what was the former province of religion, the addict can be seen as striving for a kind of salvation by accepting the sacrament of treatment under the doctrine of abstinence. For those in treatment, the wrath of an angry society is tempered. But for those who continue their illegal use of narcotics, they are to law enforcement what sinners were to Edwards' avenging God. If Puritan themes of sin, redemption, and damnation do provide the ideological metaphor for the treatment of drug users in the United States, then recovery from addiction would be the sole acceptable path to HIV prevention. Syringe exchange, to the ideological descendants of Jonathan Edwards, to follow the metaphor, would be no more acceptable than craven image worship would be to Edwards himself. Syringe exchange has indeed become a hotly debated symbolic issue. It separates those who would reduce the harm addicts are subject to by increasing access to sterile syringes from those who insist that not another inch of America be surrendered to the drug addicts and criminals who they fear threaten their version of America as it should be, irrespective of the consequences for drug users.

Contemporary American drug control policy is putatively based on the Keynesian economic model of 'supply and demand'. Enforcement attempts seek to reduce the *supply* of illicit drugs (or diversion of prescription medicines to users); and treatment and prevention efforts seek to reduce the *demand* for these substances. In order to reduce demand for illegal drugs, the United States government supports prevention activities that seek to convince non drug users not to start, and to convince or enable existing users to quit. In some instances medical treatment is offered, in others lip service is paid to the problem as in the Reagan Administration's 'Just Say No' campaign. Included in the programme of disincentives for drug users was the enactment of strict, punitive laws, minimum mandatory sentences for convicted drug offenders, and the 'zero tolerance' seizure laws. These policies permitted the seizure of property (houses, land, automobiles, boats, etc.) where banned drugs were found. In some instances amounts as small as a few cannabis seeds have been sufficient for such seizures of property. In addition to strict interdiction policies, a federally funded drug treatment system has been established. Despite substantial federal and local funding for public drug treatment, there are waiting lists – often months long – in the overwhelming majority of publicly funded drug treatment clinics in the United States. American gaols and prisons are swollen beyond capacity with drug statute violators, who account for a substantial proportion of the burgeoning prison population. In California alone, 27 per cent of all the 470,932 adult criminal arrests during 1992 were for violations of drug laws.

Neither the relationship between drug users, drug treatment, and the criminal justice system nor the zeal with which this enforcement agenda is pursued has been altered by the rapid onset of the HIV/AIDS epidemic among drug users. Contemporary American society views and treats drug users as morally corrupted, reprehensible, and disposable. This metaphor of drug users as sinners in the hands of an angry God binds the foundation of anti-narcotics laws and social policies that have determined the direction of substance abuse prevention, treatment, and interdiction activities over the past hundred years. This has resulted in jealously guarded policies that resist any efforts that might be interpreted as *enabling*, or at the very least as *tolerating*, any form of illicit drug use. For the neo-Puritan ideologues, syringe exchange is an immoral enterprise, for if drug use is a sin, then access to needles and syringes and exchange programmes enables it. Much of the resistance to syringe exchange in the United States is built upon this religious bedrock. And there is significant political support for the right-wing ideologues who oppose, restrict, and inhibit AIDS prevention programmes such as conservative Republican Senator Jesse Helms of North Carolina. At present, there are only five states that lack both needle prescription laws and paraphernalia laws. There are only two that have changed laws to permit the legal operation of syringe exchange (Connecticut and Hawaii). The major shifts in the needle prescription and drug paraphernalia laws, needed to enable broad implementation of needle and syringe exchange programmes, have failed to materialise in the vast majority of United States jurisdictions. Senator Helms has led resistance at the federal level by including language in the annual appropriations law that prohibits the use of federal funds for syringe exchange, unless the Surgeon-General first finds that syringe exchange is necessary to control the AIDS epidemic. As was seen in the reaction to Surgeon-General Elders' suggestion that marijuana be reconsidered for possible medical applications, any perceived loosening of drug laws is politically taboo. In this political environment, the likelihood that any elected or appointed official at the federal level will confront the adamant political and religious opposition to syringe exchange is not high.

RESISTANCE IN THE AFRICAN AMERICAN COMMUNITY: RELIGIOUS TIES, COMMUNITIES BESET AND THE GHOSTS OF TUSKEGEE

While there is no clear unanimity of opinion regarding syringe exchange in the African American community, there has been considerable and often vociferous opposition from some (but certainly not all) religious and secular leaders (Thomas and Quinn, 1993). Nevertheless, opposition in the African American community represents one of the roots of resistance to syringe exchange. This opposition is more complex than the ideological and moralistic objections of the (predominantly white) religious right. Over time, dialogue about the relative merits and demerits of syringe exchange has become more open, even among some community leaders and members who had once held views of extreme opposition. Three major themes have emerged from this dialogue. These are: (1) moral and religious opposition, not dissimilar to that of the evangelical right; (2) a vested interest and deep concern for the high cost of drug abuse in African American communities in human, economic, and cultural terms; and (3) mistrust of government institutions, the professionals who staff them, and health policies generated by the government. From the slave encounter through two hundred years of segregation, the road to grasping African American opposition to syringe exchange runs directly through Tuskegee, Alabama.

Throughout the United States, the African American leadership draws heavily from the churches in its community. Much of the Protestant tradition in the African American community is derived from early American missionary zeal. As such, these churches share a common root with other Protestant sects with roots in the Puritan awakening, so it is not surprising that members of these churches view drug use as immoral and essentially sinful. A more pragmatic and secular concern is that many African American communities have high rates of drug addiction. Frustration with the negative consequences of drug use in these communities is high and can stem from personal experience with close friends and relatives and/or conflicts with drug users and sellers who reside or operate in the community. Drug use, signs of drug use, and the characterisation of communities as 'high risk for drug use' are factors that can contribute to economic stagnation. Community members with livelihoods at stake object to their communities being characterised as 'high risk'. To many, this is a racist label that relegates an entire community to the economic scrap heap. Given this view, activities that abet drug users in their addiction seem, at best, misdirected since such activities do not seek to eliminate drug use and drug users from the environment. Worse, these efforts are seen by opponents as encouraging drug use. In the African American community, syringe exchange is sometimes seen as diverting resources from the fundamental economic and social problems in order to deal with the symptoms of those problems. To these opponents, spending money on syringe exchange (which does not have as its goal abstinence from drug use) when those same resources might go into drug abuse treatment can be viewed as the abandonment of African American communities to long-term patterns of crime and drug abuse. To some, needle exchange is a nonsense approach advocated by persons who live outside of the community, do not understand it, and do not care about its well-being.

The perception that syringe exchange is an idea fostered by the white majority further alienates some members of the African American community. Syringe exchange is often viewed as untested in the African American community. Its outcomes in these venues, it is argued, is unknown, and this kind of research in a living community is seen as ethically questionable and reminiscent of the Tuskegee syphilis experiment. It is in the Tuskegee syphilis experiment that we find one of the clearest symbols of the failure of the American medical establishment to protect the interests of African Americans, and one of the principal obstacles to establishing adequate HIV prevention programmes in the black community. The cry 'Tuskegee' evokes memories of government-sponsored racism and medical cruelty in the name of medical research. Why should syringe exchange experiments be any different?

The Tuskegee syphilis experiment was begun in 1932 and was finally terminated only after press coverage in 1972 forced the issue to the floor of the United States Senate. This infamous project was conducted by the US Public Health Service (including members of the US Centers for Disease Control) who ostensibly sought to learn more about the natural history of syphilis in black males by observing syphilis-infected men over the course of their lifetimes without treating them for the disease. Government health officials selected a poor, predominantly African American county in the rural South for this natural history study. Without the benefit of informed consent, 399 men with syphilis were enrolled. As a condition of participation, treatment was withheld. This condition was observed throughout the life of the study, even after the discovery that penicillin could provide effective treatment for syphilis. As an incentive, participants were promised a free annual medical check-up for life, a nominal cash payment, and a free burial. In 1972, some forty years after the study had begun, the Associated Press broke the story that would end the Tuskegee experiment. Some press reports placed the number of study participants who had died of syphilis or its complications at 28 men and perhaps as many as 100 (Jones, 1993).

The study was conducted under government auspices, in the contemporary era, and with no reasonable regard for the rights and well-being of those men who trusted the government physicians who conducted the experiment. The Tuskegee syphilis experiment has left two important legacies. The first is the codification of modern ethical standards for the conduct of research involving human subjects. The second was a fresh wind under the smouldering mistrust of white institutions in the African American community. After Tuskegee, why indeed should blacks trust outsiders conducting health research or experimentation with human subjects?

In the politics of syringe exchange, Tuskegee is merely one example of the betrayal of African Americans by American medical and government institutions. Preventable and curable diseases such as tuberculosis are resurgent in African American communities, which continue to suffer high rates of infectious diseases, infant mortality, malnutrition, and illiteracy that are more on a par with Third World countries than with those of their white American counterparts. Emblematic of the disjuncture in world views of many African American community members and public health professionals is the failure of these professionals to take seriously a question that is asked in earnest in the African American community: 'Is AIDS genocide?'

In 1990, 35 per cent of 979 black church members in five United States' cities agreed with the statement 'I believe that AIDS is a form of genocide against the black race.' Another 30 per cent reported that they were unsure (Thomas and Quinn, 1993). In essence, AIDS, like the Tuskegee syphilis experiment, has become a metaphor for genocidal fears among African Americans. During the mid 1980s, ethnographic research among drug users in San Francisco revealed that many IDUs believed AIDS was a government plot. Many persist in their belief that HIV is the product of a government laboratory. Some believed that it was a disease designed to kill gays and drug users. The views of these IDUs reflected concerns that are not uncommon in the African American community.

POLITICAL RESISTANCE: ELECTORAL POLITICS AND THE NON-VOTING DRUG USER

Through all of the debate, trial programmes, and slow movement on the syringe exchange issue in America, IDUs have been, both individually and as a group, the silent object of this ferment. There are few segments of contemporary society that have been more excluded, vilified, and persecuted. At the root of this vulnerability is the fact that IDUs pose no threat as a unified political force. There are no political action committees or lobbyists in

Washington or state capitals to represent the self-perceived interests of IDUs. They are a highly unpopular group. They occupy the lowest rungs in the status hierarchy, even among the 'underclass'. Given their high vulnerability and unpopularity, the exploitation of drug users by ambitious political entrepreneurs has become something of a tradition in the United States.[2]

There can be little doubt that injection drug use represents a serious health risk for those so engaged. But this health risk is closely linked to enforcement efforts that seek to eradicate the non-medical use of unsanctioned psychoactive drugs through a system of harsh disincentives. These policies have greatly increased the health risks that would otherwise be restricted to the pharmacological properties of the drugs used. The risks of infection with viral hepatitis and HIV are raised enormously by restricting access to the disposable, single-use syringe, an instrument that was developed for the express purpose of reducing the spread of infectious diseases. While the moralisation/criminalisation of drug use and drug users may discourage use for some, for those it fails to discourage, it punishes. Often this punishment is a pitiless persecution, and a willingness to allow exposure to otherwise preventable and often fatal illness. Those who are physiologically addicted, or for whom the compulsion to inject drugs is greater than the perceived disincentives or ability to stop, society places at grave risk. If our experience of drug treatment, drug prevention, and drug enforcement has taught us anything, it is that there will always be a sizeable minority who will continue to use drugs under even the most draconian threats of punishment and the most dire predictions of disease. As drugs have been demonised and drug users vilified, it has become possible to view drug users as the authors of their own condition, and to punish them severely for their 'immorality', their 'weakness', and their 'sinful' attributes. As the inevitable conclusion, drug users become the target of persecution. Through this process, society hopes to define itself by what it will not tolerate. Unchampioned and unpopular, drug users are easy scapegoats and the frequent target of elected politicians who hope to garner votes by playing on the fear of drugs and drug users. The history of American drug control policy is well-populated by persons who have sought to salvage political and bureaucratic careers through the campaigns against drugs and drug users (Musto, 1973; Epstein, 1977).

The effect of political expediency on social and health policies, including those associated with AIDS, should not be underestimated. It is here that the door to a more humanistic and rational approach to social problems related to drug use is barred. And the equation is simple: votes equals office. In general, American politicians, political appointees, and political bureaucrats, not health professionals, hold the keys to the door of health policy. While one might reasonably argue that to deny drug addicts access to sterile syringes in the midst of a virulent, blood-borne epidemic is impractical and unethical, one might also argue that to permit syringe exchange, given the religious and ideological opposition to it, is politically maladroit.

An example of this can be seen in the history of syringe exchange legislation in California. In 1992, a non-binding referendum was passed by the voters of San Francisco to permit syringe exchange. The same year the San Francisco Health Commission passed a resolution supporting syringe exchange, the County Board of Supervisors also passed a resolution supporting syringe exchange.[3] Following months of hearings on the subject, both the upper and lower houses of the California state legislature passed bills making syringe exchange legal. Under California law, the Governor was not required to approve or sign the bill for it to pass into law. Nevertheless, Republican Governor Pete Wilson, yielding to pressure from the Bush Administration's Office of Narcotic Drug Control Policy (ONDCP), vetoed the bill at the eleventh hour. Governor Wilson cited an ONDCP white paper taking the position that scientific evaluation had failed to provide conclusive results that HIV could be halted through syringe exchange, and that such programmes serve to undermine progress on drug prevention initiatives.

One year later, in 1993, after more hearings, both houses of the California legislature once again approved a bill making syringe exchange legal in counties where the health officer deemed programmes desirable. Indeed, some syringe exchange advocates had hoped that Wilson, widely held to be a moderate Republican, would permit the bill to become law, particularly in light of recent research and due to a more supportive environment in Washington. Gone was the Bush Administration whose drug czar, Martinez, had issued orders to Wilson the previous year to hold to the party line. But Governor Wilson's popularity was slipping in the polls. Drug users are not a voting bloc, and the liberal vote had always been against Wilson. What the Governor needed to do was to shore up his rapidly eroding base of support among conservative Republicans, many with close ties to the religious right. Only hours before the legislation enabling syringe exchange would have become law in the most populated state in the United States, Governor Pete Wilson once again executed his veto.

Conservative ideologues like Wilson make two principal arguments in their opposition to syringe exchange. The first is that it will not reduce risk behaviour or HIV infection rates. The second is that effective syringe exchange is undesirable because removing negative consequences associated with drug abuse (e.g. AIDS) will undermine drug abuse prevention efforts and out-comes. While none of the studies published to date has found such a negative effect, there is enormous sentiment on this point. The findings of a study of syringe exchange commissioned by the US Centers for Disease and Prevention (Lurie *et al.*, 1993), which concluded that syringe exchange was a benign and potentially useful AIDS prevention stratagem, were presented to the

Governor weeks before the deadline for his veto. Governor Wilson dismissed the findings of this study on the following grounds:

> Critics of the needle exchange programme point out that this ... data does not amount to clear evidence that in those areas where needle exchange programmes have been undertaken, a demonstrated reduction in HIV transmission has in fact occurred.

> (Wilson, 1993)

Here Governor Wilson claims that syringe exchange does not work. But also in his 1993 veto message, Wilson reveals his fear that syringe exchange does work, and that its utility in reducing new HIV infections is an undesirable outcome, since reduction of negative consequences of drug use may result in conversions of otherwise righteous young people to the sinful ranks of drug users:

> In blunt terms, is it worth reducing the risk of infection to intravenous drug users at potentially far greater cost of undermining all our other preventive anti-drug efforts and suffering as a result an enormous increase in the number of young people who make a wrong choice that leads to an enormous increase in addicts?

> If we are going to demand that young people exercise personal responsibility, if you say that *they must suffer the consequences of their personal choices*, what are they to think when in the next breath we give formal sanction to a project which facilitates drug use?

> I have not made lightly the decision to withhold my signature. I have done so fully mindful that by some estimates there are as many as 400,000 active intravenous drug users in California exposing themselves, their sexual partners, and future children to HIV ... But the choice I am compelled to make is for prevention of tomorrow's addicts, and the avoidance of all the waste, heartbreak and tragedy that flow from drug use.

> (Wilson, 1993; emphasis added)

Governor Wilson, in his veto language, evokes the images of America's Puritan past. At issue is government complicity in a plan that would actually reduce the risk of acquiring a fatal and incurable disease from drug abuse. So important is the maintenance of this threat that the Governor is willing to write off 400,000 Californians, their non drug using sexual partners, and any children they may have. No elected politician would ever write off 400,000 votes unless he or she believed they were irretrievably lost to non-participation, otherwise committed, or overpowered by a much larger constituency. Bear in mind that the road to the White House for two relatively recent Republican presidents (Nixon and Reagan) ran directly through the Governor's mansion in Sacramento. Both of these presidents took strong anti-drug stances and increased the punishments for drug users.

In this example we see one of the principal roots of resistance to syringe exchange in America. The political influence of the religious right, and the modern metaphor of the drug user as sinner. It is important not only that drug users be punished, but that this punishment be terrible and public so as to dissuade others.

SQUABBLING OVER PARADIGMS

Given this set of religious, political, and historical factors, concern over AIDS has failed to produce a fundamental shift in the underlying ideology that guides substance abuse policy in the United States. Drug users remain to contemporary America the social equivalent of heretics and sinners to Puritan New England. At best, IDUs are seen as the authors of their own conditions and are considered highly undesirable and disposable. While other Western countries may share a similar cultural, linguistic, and/or religious heritage, none has America's unique intersection of ideological and ethnic influences and considerations. Yet the United States is not alone in its difficulty in resolving public health dilemmas arising from an abhorrence of drug abuse.

Unfortunately, the need for a war on AIDS seems irreconcilable with the existing war on drug users. The keys to a more rational and productive set of health and social policies for IDUs remain illusive. Yet there has been a slow-moving change. During 1993, the US Centers for Disease Control released a report which concluded that syringe exchange was a worthwhile AIDS prevention strategy (Lurie et al., 1993). Also during 1993, the National Institute on Drug Abuse lifted its ban on research into syringe exchange and released a grant announcement soliciting research proposals that examine the issue of syringe exchange. In 1993, the National Academy of Sciences and Institute of Medicine began an examination of syringe exchange as a means of HIV prevention (National Academy of Science, 1994). Critics, however, continue to dismiss the results of these studies, at times without reading them (Associated Press, 1994). As with the veto of California's needle exchange legislation, these critics voice concerns that syringe exchange will undermine drug prevention efforts. Yet there exist no published data to support this fear. Critics also point to the absence of controlled studies which demonstrate conclusively that syringe exchange reduces HIV infection rates. Despite the preponderance of evidence in support of the usefulness of syringe exchange, there are methodological weaknesses in virtually all existing studies of syringe exchange. This should surprise no one, since there are few, if any, flawless studies of anything in the scientific literature.

The ideal experimental design for demonstrating intervention effectiveness is the so-called *clinical trial*. The clinical trial is the basis for evaluation of certain surgical or drug-based interventions, primarily in clinical or laboratory settings (Friedman, L. M. et al., 1985). Some critics steadfastly persist in their insistence that a clinical trial of syringe exchange efficacy be conducted before approval of syringe exchange be granted. Of course, it is impossible to conduct such a clinical trial if syringe exchange is not allowed. But even where syringe exchange is legal, the clinical trial presents so many problems for assessing behavioural intervention in community settings that it is doubtful such a study will ever be completed.

In such a design, HIV seronegative IDUs would be assigned at random to one of two cohorts: one with access to syringe exchange and one without such access. Members of both cohorts would be followed over time and contacted at, say, six-month intervals for interviews and blood specimens. If after some period of time (say, two or three years of follow-up), the syringe exchange group had significantly fewer serconversions for HIV than the control group, then cause and effect could be established.

But there are major problems associated with this approach. First, such a design does not, and could not, account for *sexual* transmission of HIV. Sexual transmission would have to be *held constant*. In the ideal design, no participants would have intercourse with an infected person. This, of course, is impossible to monitor in the real world. A weaker design might use self-reported data on sexual activity as *covariates* in statistical analyses, but this approach too is highly problematic, since self-reports might not be accurate, or if accurate, the HIV status of the sexual partner(s) would be difficult or impossible to confirm. Second, one might reasonably expect *contamination effects*, which would bias the study in the direction of a negative result. This would occur if, for example, friends, lovers, or other close associates were assigned to different groups. Persons with exchange privileges might assist their friends by providing clean syringes to members of the non-exchange group, thereby inadvertently foiling the study design. Should this occur, subjects who were actually receiving clean syringes from the exchange would be misclassified, and the results biased in the direction of showing no difference between study groups.

There is also the problem of sample size. Given relatively modest rates of HIV seroincidence among heterosexual IDUs in most United States' venues, a very large sample would have to be drawn. The lower the rate of new HIV infections, the greater the sample size would have to be to meet the statistical power requirement. The cost of conducting such a study could easily exceed $1.5 million per year for several years. Cost would depend primarily upon the size of the cohorts required to meet the statistical power requirements of the experiment. This number would in turn be determined by the rate of new HIV infections (incidence) occurring in the population studied (Meinert, 1986). The higher the incidence rate, the smaller the sample size requirement. Very few sites in the United States could meet the criteria of having a large population of IDUs and high enough HIV seroincidence to make such a study feasible, and in fewer still would the laws permit such a study to be conducted. Consequently, critics of syringe exchange insist on an unrealistic standard for its evaluation.

In the case of syringe exchange, strict adherence to experimental standards of proof may not be practical, feasible, scientifically appropriate or ethically defensible (Gerber *et al.*, 1994).

It is worth noting that this experimental burden of proof has not been placed on other health interventions that are based on studies of the type already used to evaluate syringe exchange. Laws which ban smoking in public places, and voluntary guidelines such as those relating to reduced intake of fatty foods, use of automobile seatbelts, and motorcycle crash helmets, are not based on clinical trials research. Rather, they are typically based on retrospective case control studies. In this research design, persons with a disease (or injury) condition are compared to persons without the condition. Possible environmental, biological, and behavioural factors are considered in statistical analyses to distinguish factors that are associated with diseased individuals (Armstrong *et al.*, 1992). Through these methods, much of what is known about the relationship of cigarette smoking to lung disease, fatty diets to cardiac and circulatory disease, and exposure to asbestos to asbestosis is based on the case control study. Following this analytic paradigm, our own study of needle sharing in San Francisco examined needle sharers with non needle sharers and found that the more often IDUs used the needle exchange in San Francisco, the less likely they were to report recent needle sharing (Watters *et al.*, 1994). While case control studies are enormously useful in identifying risk factors, they are limited in their application in the evaluation of social programmes. Nevertheless, under the existing legal, political, and funding environment, such studies represent one of few feasible alternatives for gaining evaluative perspectives on syringe exchange programmes.

In refusing to accept existing data, opponents of syringe exchange use an argument employed by the tobacco industry in defending the production and marketing of cigarettes for the last several decades. The tobacco industry insists that case control studies cannot *prove* that cigarette smoking *causes* respiratory disease, only that cigarette smoking may be a *risk factor* in such illness. This is a subtle distinction, to be sure. The tobacco industry and their lobbyists at the American Tobacco Institute point out the absence of *controlled studies* (clinical trials). Opponents of syringe exchange use the same logic, and insist on unrealistic and unfeasible standards for evaluating outcomes. In dismissing existing studies, resistance to syringe exchange sets criteria for evaluation that have not been required of a dizzying array of social programmes, surgical interventions, and drug-based therapies. Of course, what is needed is the political will to make the public health decisions which hold out the greatest likelihood of reducing continued HIV contagion. Politics is, however, a short-sighted profession. Its collective vision rarely extends past the next election. Consequently, resistance to syringe exchange in the United States continues to hold sway.

EPILOGUE

On 30 September 1994, Governor Pete Wilson of California vetoed, for the third consecutive year, legislation that would have permitted county health officials the option of including syringe exchange in their portfolio of AIDS prevention efforts. Once again Governor Wilson cited the need to enforce accountability for personal choices, the lack of conclusive proof that syringe exchange reduces HIV, and the fear that syringe exchange would encourage drug abuse.

ACKNOWLEDGEMENTS

The author wishes to thank Michelle Aldrich, Ricky N. Bluthenthal, John G. Fisher, Stephen Fitzhenry, and Starley B. Shade for their contributions.

NOTES

1 Witches were put to death in colonial America. At Salem, Massachusetts, during a period May through October 1692, twenty-seven people were arrested for witchcraft. Nineteen were hanged, and one was pressed to death by having rocks placed on him. In most instances the corpses were burned. Cotton Mather (1663–1728) was a Puritan theologian who contributed to the witchcraft hysteria through his writings which supported the persecution of witches.
2 The history of American narcotics control policy includes the public opinion campaigns of Admiral Pearson Hobson, Harry J. Anslinger, Governor Nelson Rockerfeller (New York) and Presidents Richard M. Nixon and Ronald Reagan. Epstein (1977) profiles the manipulation of substance abuse policy for political purposes from Hobson through to Nixon.
3 It should be pointed out that San Francisco tends to be significantly more liberal in its voting proclivities than California as a whole, which tends to reflect a large conservative constituency.

REFERENCES

Armstrong, B. K., White, E., and Saracci, R. (1992) *Principles of Exposure Measurement in Epidemiology*, New York: Oxford University Press.
Associated Press (1994) 'Studies support needle exchanges: addicts readily shift from dirty syringes – a link to spread of AIDS', *Washington Post*, Wednesday, January 12, 1994, A3.
Buzolic, A. (1988). *Needle and Syringe Availability and AIDS Prevention: Modifications of Existing Legislation*, Queensland, Australia: Australia Ministerial Task Force on Drug Strategy.
Des Jarlais, D. C., Hagan, H., Purchase, D., Reid, T., and Friedman, S. R. (1989) 'Safer injection among participants in the first North American syringe exchange program', in *Abstracts from the 5th International Conference on AIDS, Montreal, Canada*, p. 58, International Development Research Centre.
Dole, V. P. and Nyswander, M. E. (1965) 'A medical treatment for diacetyl-morphine (heroin) addiction'. *Journal of the American Medical Association*, 193, 80.
—— (1967) 'Heroin addiction: a metabolic disease', *Archives of Internal Medicine*, 120, 119.

Dole, V. P., Nyswander, M. E., and Warner, A. (1968) 'Successful treatment of 750 criminal addicts', *Journal of the American Medical Association*, 206, 2708–2711.

Edwards, J. (1741) 'Sinners in the Hands of an Angry God,' in O. Winslow (ed.) *Jonathan Edwards: Basic Writings*, New York, NY: Penguin Books.

Epstein, E. J. (1977) *Agency of Fear*, New York: G.P. Putnam's Sons.

Francis, D. P. (1992) 'Toward a comprehensive HIV prevention program for the CDC and the nation', *Journal of the American Medical Association*, 268, 1444–1447.

Friedman, L. M., Furberg, C. D., and DeMetz, D. L. (1985) *Fundamentals of Clinical Trials*, (2nd edn), Littleton, MA: PSG Publishing.

Friedman, S. R., Des Jarlais, D C., Wenston J., WHO Collaborative Study Group (1994) 'New injectors remain at high risk for HIV infection', in *Tenth International Conference on AIDS*, Yokohama, Japan.

Gerber, R. A., Campbell, C. H., Dillon, B. A., and Holtgrave, D. R. (1994) 'Evaluating behavioural interventions: need for randomized controlled trials', *Journal of the American Medical Association*, 271, 1317–1318.

Hart, G. J., Carvell, A. L. M., Woodward, N., Johnson, A. M., Williams, P., and Parry, J. V. (1989) 'Evaluation of needles exchange in central London: behaviour change and anti-HIV status over one year', *AIDS*, 3, 261–265.

Hartgers, C., Buning, E. C., van Santen, G. W., Verster, A. D., and Coutinho, R. A. (1989) 'The impact of the needle and syringe exchange programme in Amsterdam in injecting risk behaviour', *AIDS*, 3, 571–576.

Husak, D. N. (1992) *Drugs and Rights*, New York: Cambridge University Press.

Jones, J. H. (1992) 'The Tuskegee Legacy. AIDS and the Black Community', *Hastings Center Report*, 6, 38–40.

Kaplan, E. H. and Heimer, R. (1992) 'HIV prevalence among intravenous drug users: model-based estimates from New Haven's legal needle exchange', *Journal of Acquired Immune Deficiency Syndromes*, 5,163–169.

Lattin, D. (1988) 'Chicago meeting: religious scholars chart fear of AIDS', *San Francisco Chronicle*, November 23, A7.

Ljunberg, B., Christensson, B., Tuning, K., Anderson, B., Landvall, B., Lyndberg, M., Zall-Friberg, A. C. (1991) 'HIV prevention among injecting drug users: three years' experience from a syringe exchange program in Sweden', *Journal of Acquired Immune Deficiency Syndromes*, 4,890–895.

Lurie, P., Reingold, A. L., Bowser, B., Chen, D., Foley, J., Guydish, J., Kahn, J. G., Lane, S., and Sorensen, J. (1993) *The Public Health Impact of Needle Exchange Programs in the United States and Abroad, Volume 1*, Atlanta, GA: US Centers for Disease Control and Prevention.

Meinert, C. L. (1986) *Clinical Trials: Design, Conduct, and Analysis*, New York: Oxford University Press.

Musto, D. F. (1973) *The American Disease: The Origins of Narcotic Control*, New Haven, CT: Yale University Press.

National Academy of Sciences (1994) *Proceedings: Workshop on Needle Exchange and Bleach Distribution Programs*, Washington D.C.: National Academy Press.

Nelson, K.E., Vlahov, D., Cohn, S. *et al.* (1991) 'Human immunodeficiency virus infection in diabetic intravenous drug users', *Journal of the American Medical Association*, 255, 2259–2261.

Purchase, D., Hagan, H., Des Jarlais, D. C., and Reid, T. (1989) 'Historical account of the Tacoma syringe exchange', in *Abstracts from the 5th International Conference on AIDS, Montreal, Canada*, p. 771, International Development Research Centre.

Pye, M., Kapila, M., Buckley, G., and Cunningham, D. (1989) 'A comparative study of local AIDS programs in the United Kingdom', in *Abstracts from the 5th International Conference on AIDS, Montreal, Canada*, p. 841, International Development Research Centre.

Smith, J. E. (1992) *Jonathan Edwards: Puritan, Preacher, Philosopher*, Notre Dame, IN: University of Notre Dame Press.

Stimson, G. V. (1989) 'Syringe-exchange programmes for injecting drug users', *AIDS*, 3, 253–260.

Thomas, S. B. and Quinn, S. C. (1993) 'Understanding the attitudes of black Americans', in J. Stryker and M. D. Smith (eds), *Dimensions of HIV Prevention: Needle Exchange*, Menlo Park, CA: The Henry J. Kaiser Family Foundation.

US Centers for Disease Control and Prevention (1994) *HIV/AIDS Surveillance Report: US HIV and AIDS cases reported through June 1994*, Atlanta, GA: US Department of Health and Human Sciences.

van den Hoek, J. A., van Haastrecht, H. J., and Coutinho, R. A. (1989) 'Risk reduction among intravenous drug users in Amsterdam under the influence of AIDS', *American Journal of Public Health*, 10, 1355–1357.

Watters, J. K., Estilo, M. J., Clark, G. L., and Lorvick, J. J. (1994) 'Syringe and needle exchange as HIV/AIDS prevention for injection drug users', *Journal of the American Medical Association*, 271, 115–120.

Wilson, P. (1993) Letter from Governor Pete Wilson to the members of the California Assembly, regarding Assembly Bill No. 260, Sacramento, CA.

Chapter 4

AIDS prevention and drug policy
Dilemmas in the local environment

Richard Hartnoll and Dagmar Hedrich

A wide variety of interventions aim to develop community-based health promotion and AIDS prevention amongst drug injectors and others who may be involved in high-risk behaviours. These include outreach, low-threshold crisis centres, methadone programmes, needle exchanges, and peer or street education projects. This chapter takes a broader perspective, and looks at how the wider environment affects the implementation and impact of these various local interventions.

The wider environment can be characterised in terms of different though interwoven spheres, for example the physical environment, the political and economic environment, the human and social environment, the policy environment, and the service environment. In each sphere, the present situation is the most recent stage in a dynamic process of conflict, cooperation and compromise between different actors and interests.

The emphasis in this chapter is on the local level, and in particular, on the city. However, in each of the spheres listed above, the wider national and sometimes international context has important effects on the local situation. A further important dimension of the broader environment is that of various audiences, such as the international community, national authorities, public opinion and the media. The reactions, or anticipated reactions, of these audiences may have a profound effect on actions taken within each sphere, both at macro- and at micro-level.

It is not possible to develop here a comprehensive analysis of how all dimensions of the environment might affect community-based interventions. Rather, some key points are selected and examined, based on the concrete example of Frankfurt.

FRANKFURT

Frankfurt is a relatively small city of 650,000 inhabitants, though the number of people in the city increases to over a million during working hours. It is situated in the state (*Land*) of Hessen and is the commercial, social and cultural centre for a much larger population living in surrounding towns and cities. Over the past 30 years there has been a major shift from traditional manufacturing to financial, service and high-tech industries. During the 1980s, Frankfurt grew as an international commercial and banking centre, and supported an extensive development of cultural facilities. In parallel with these changes, many of the more wealthy moved out of the city. This process led to the movement of poorer people, including immigrants, into areas of the inner city, to a growth in the importance of the city centre for business, shopping, consumption and leisure, and to an increased priority for transport links to the city (private car and train for commuters; motorways, train and airport for business). Today, as a major commercial centre, Frankfurt is at the hub of a network of communication, trade and transport links at local, national and European level. Traditionally an SPD (Social Democrat) city, it was governed by the CDU (conservatives) from 1977 until March 1989, when an SPD/Green coalition was elected.

THE EMERGENCE OF AIDS: CONSTRAINTS ON THE RESPONSE

In the second half of the 1980s, Frankfurt, like many cities, was confronted with rising concern about HIV and AIDS. Over the same period, the number of IDUs in the city rose sharply (this mainly involved heroin and occurred in other parts of Germany as well). Anxiety about the possible consequences of a spread of HIV amongst drug users and the partly overlapping population of prostitutes intensified the debate over drug policy and over how to minimise the dangers presented by HIV.

As in other countries, the options discussed in Germany included interventions aimed at reaching drug injectors, for example through crisis centres or outreach, and at developing preventive measures, for example methadone or syringe exchange. However, unlike countries such as Britain or the Netherlands, but like countries such as France or Belgium, there were serious structural and cultural obstacles to implementing many of these interventions. Thus, federal drug policy over the preceding years had been intolerant, emphasising repression of users and (often coercive) drug-free treatment. German legislation prohibited the prescription of methadone, the medical establishment and the Ministry of Health were opposed to drug substitution, and the main form of treatment was provided by therapeutic communities (after detoxification in a psychiatric ward).

There were counselling centres, usually run by non-governmental organisations (NGOs) or religious organisations and staffed by social workers and psychologists, but they had little tradition or experience of street work. Furthermore, their client- or family-oriented case approach, and their training in therapy and counselling, meant that they were often reluctant to change how they worked or to implement measures like methadone or syringe exchange which appeared to accept continued drug use or injecting.

A further obstacle to changes in treatment and service provision was the medical insurance companies, who remained unwilling to accept as 'treatment' anything that was not defined in narrow, medical terms of detoxification. Drug-free treatment in therapeutic communities was considered as rehabilitation and was paid for by pension schemes, but they refused to extend this to methadone or other harm-reduction approaches.

As in most countries, drug addicts were stigmatised and rejected. However, from the late 1970s and throughout the 1980s, the (conservative) national government, especially the Ministry of the Interior, adopted an increasingly repressive and militaristic tone concerning the war on heroin (echoing the terminology of the fight against terrorism that was also preoccupying them at the time). The 1980s saw the tightening of legislation (Opiates Act 1981) and the scapegoating of addiction as an infectious disease, initially at federal level, subsequently in the *Länder*.

Thus when AIDS emerged as an issue in the mid-1980s, the attitudes of politicians, professionals and public alike were highly negative and moralistic. With few exceptions, physicians and psychiatrists were reluctant to treat addicts or provide health care; the police, prosecutors and courts followed a severe and punitive line; community leaders and the public wanted drugs and drug addiction removed from view; and addicts were often rejected by their families and local communities.

These elements exist in all modern societies, but were particularly marked in the historical and cultural context described here. That context, and the structural constraints outlined above, meant that there was little space left for drug addicts in the Germany of the mid-1980s, and that there was limited room for manoeuvre to develop policies and interventions to prevent AIDS and reduce harm arising from drug use.

The process of meeting this challenge, and the dilemmas that arose, are discussed through an historical account of the evolution of drug addiction, drug policy and AIDS prevention in Frankfurt. The key local players are drawn from different spheres: law enforcement (police, prosecutor), politics (mayor, councillors, opposition, local elections), city administrations (Health, Social Affairs, Drugs Policy Division), non-governmental organisations, commerce (business, shops and banks), residents and commuters. The physical structure of the city, the transport links, the public space, the housing situation and socio-demographic distribution of the population were all important factors. Beyond the city boundaries, the policies of the State of Hessen and other German *Länder*, of nearby cities, of the Federal Government, and of the medical insurance companies also played significant roles.

BEFORE AIDS: THE DRUG SCENE AND RESPONSES TO IT

A visible drug scene first developed in Frankfurt in 1967–68 in a park at the upper end of Taunusanlage, in front of the Old Opera. At this time drug use mainly involved cannabis and was associated with students, political protest and other cultural changes that were taking place amongst the youth of many countries.

In the 1970s, the nature and structure of the drug scene changed (Noller, 1991). The student scene split into 'cannabis rebels' and serious political activists who rejected drugs. New groups of users appeared, including middle-class 'drop-outs' and especially lower-class adolescents who were released following the closure of foster homes. Early in the 1970s other drugs, including opiates, were also used. By the mid-1970s, youth unemployment was rising, squatting and self-governing communes had expanded, and violent youth gangs from working-class areas emerged. Heroin became available and whole groups started injecting, including the youth gangs, amongst whom heroin use was a symbol of 'toughness'. A surge in the number of drug-related deaths led to increased concern about drug taking.

Responses to drug use became more repressive over this period, especially in the latter half of the decade. However, until 1979 the open drug scene, which was not very large, was tolerated in the park through informal understandings between police, city officials and the users, though police controls increased at the end of the 1970s. Those who were involved refer to mutual self-support between users in the scene.

In 1979, a report commissioned by the city government (which changed from SPD to CDU in 1977) concluded that Frankfurt had a negative image. This was the start of a process of modernisation and development of the image of Frankfurt as an international city. The policy aimed to attract business, services and high-tech industries, to revitalise the city centre, and to develop high-profile cultural facilities and activities.

In 1980 it was decided to close down the open drug scene in the park. The police were opposed, because it was easier to control the situation when it was visible and in one place. However, the Mayor prevailed, supported by local political and commercial interests, and encouraged by a Federal Government which was waging an increasingly ideological war against drugs.

The drug scene was then chased around the city by the police from one open space to the next, until by 1981 it had become largely established in and around the main station. At the time, this was an underdeveloped area with cheap hotels, a poor, multi-ethnic population, and a tradition of prostitution that had grown since the Second World War. The open drug scene was probably allowed to develop there because it did not threaten any powerful interests. From a police perspective, it was perhaps seen as preferable to contain the scene in one area. Some see it as deliberate segregation, a way of managing the use of the space in a city and of regulating social problems. A small scene continued to be visible in the park from time to time.

The decision to close the open scene, and the subsequent pursuit of addicts around different parts of Frankfurt, led to a debate in the early 1980s about the need for social help and outreach, since increased repression and criminalisation meant that addicts were unwilling to go to traditional services. For example, applying an existing law, addicts picked up by the police were taken to a judge and a doctor, who at times were situated in a car near the open scene (one form of outreach!). This could lead to immediate enforced short-term admission to psychiatric hospital, followed by the possibility of long-term compulsory treatment in a psychiatric clinic 50 kilometres from Frankfurt which had been a concentration and execution camp for the psychologically handicapped in the last war. Apart from this clinic, there were a few counselling facilities and therapeutic communities run by NGOs in or around the city, but these dealt with relatively few drug users.

The first half of the 1980s saw the emergence of small but articulate groups who criticised the prevailing policy and pressed for alternative approaches. The first outreach project was set up near the main station in 1982 (though closed in 1988 due to internal rifts). In 1983, a Junkie Union was formed, but lasted only a few months, mainly due to the pressures of survival under conditions of continual police control. A telephone helpline was also set up by a new NGO in the same year. In 1985, another outreach project was started by an independent NGO (AIDS-Hilfe). In 1984–85, research projects on self-recovery began, reflecting the emergence of an alternative perspective that saw drug addiction as a stage in a process of identity formation within a societal context, rather than as a state of disease (Kindermann *et al.*, 1989; Schneider and Happel, 1987).

From the mid-1980s, the city started to 'clean up' the image of the station area. Space was needed for commercial development and further expansion of business in the city. The growing number of people coming into Frankfurt (commuters and visitors) meant that the drug trade and prostitution were increasingly seen as a negative image at the 'entrance to the city'. There were also many complaints from shops in and around the station precinct. However, the attempt to expel drug users from the station area did not really succeed, largely because of the mounting pressure of other factors that were outside the control of the city authorities or police.

From 1987, after a period of relative stability since the early 1980s, the prevalence of heroin use and addiction started to increase in many parts of Germany, including Frankfurt and nearby cities. The availability of heroin rose and prices fell. The fact that Frankfurt was a major commercial and financial centre with excellent local, national and international transport and communication links was very likely an important factor in stimulating the heroin market in the city.

At the same time, the repression and scapegoating of addicts had increased in other parts of Hessen (where the conservatives had replaced the SPD in 1985) and in other more conservative neighbouring *Länder* such as Bavaria and Baden-Württemberg. For example, the drug scenes in Darmstadt, Wiesbaden and Hanau were broken up by the police. This added to the influx of addicts into Frankfurt, many of them without accommodation.

The characteristics of the station itself were also an important factor. It was the central connection point with other towns and cities, and in a key position linking different parts of the city. There was a large amount of anonymous space within and near the station, with a complex of different levels, shopping precinct, car parks, corridors, stairways and entrances. The failure to expel the open drug scene from the station area was thus in large part because there was little other space for the growing number of addicts to go where they would be tolerated. However, as the numbers grew, and policing in the station area intensified, drug scenes expanded in other open spaces, notably the Taunusanlage park, surrounded by the major banks of Frankfurt, not far from where it had started in 1967–68.

By 1990, an estimated 6–8,000 heroin addicts were supplied by the Frankfurt market (though not all at one time). Over half, and in the open scene at least two-thirds, were from outside of Frankfurt. Their state of health was increasingly poor, and the number of drug-related deaths was rising (from 31 in 1985 to 108 in 1990). Apprehension amongst local citizens about the growing visibility of drug injecting and about drug related crime was also increasing.

AFTER AIDS: DRUG POLICY DEVELOPMENTS

The situation described above coincided with increasing concern about HIV and AIDS, and growing pressure to examine alternative approaches, including reports from the Federal AIDS Commission (Deutscher Bundestag, 1988). In 1987, federal policy changed, and the Ministry of Health started to talk about reducing stigmatisation, to suggest that injecting should not be used as a reason for repression, and to encourage the sale of syringes, needle exchange, outreach and other measures to reduce health risks.

Drug policy in Frankfurt, though not in surrounding Hessen, started to change in 1988, the year before local elections, and the debate about alternatives to repression intensified. The police and city government were criticised for pursuing a policy that increased the risks of HIV (e.g. by continually moving addicts on or by confiscating syringes) and gave too little emphasis to the development of services. At the same time, public anxiety about citizens' safety was rising, as were demands that something be done about 'the problem'. However, the police too were starting to wonder whether they could control the situation purely through repression. Despite increased pressure, the scene around the station remained, and in the Taunusanlage was growing.

In the autumn of 1988, a drug coordination group was established involving regular meetings of the police, prosecutor and city health and welfare authorities. At first, more attention was given to questions of public order and safety, though subsequently the balance changed.

In March 1989, the Green/SPD coalition won the city elections. Their platform included developing an alternative approach to drug addiction in the city. In September, a Drug Policy Division (DPD) was set up under the responsibility of the Councillor for Women and Health (Green party) who also took over as Chair of the Monday policy coordination meetings. This group (the *Montagsrunde*) still continues to meet every Monday morning and has played a central role in developing drug policy in Frankfurt. In addition to the Monday group, weekly Friday meetings were started involving the DPD, NGOs and the police, to discuss cooperation on more practical issues.

Statement of the new drug policy

The new city government and the DPD set about the task of developing and implementing a new and distinctive drug policy. A final statement of the Monday policy group 'To Live with Drug Addicts' was agreed in April 1991 by the City Council (Frankfurt am Main, 1991b) after consultation with the political parties. The starting point for this statement was the recognition that:

> The attempt to eliminate drugs and drug use from our culture has failed. It seems probable that in the future we will have to continue to live with drugs and drug users. Instead of denying this fact, we should create the conditions that enable the reduction of risks, limit damage, and reduce suffering.

The debate on drug policy, and the development of new initiatives, pre-dated the founding of the DPD, and continued to evolve and change after this 'final statement' was agreed. However, it was an important landmark which represented one of the few explicit and systematic attempts to create a consensus around a drug policy based on harm reduction involving a city administration, health and social services, police and prosecutor, NGOs, school administration, and local political, commercial and public interests.

The central element of the policy was that reduction of harm for drug users and protection of citizens were seen as equally important. For the former, emphasis was placed on health and social policy measures; for the latter, repressive measures were to focus on the illegal trade and on protecting citizens from its consequences. Other dimensions concerned recommendations for initiatives at the level of the *Land* (Hessen) and the Federal Government, especially for reducing restrictions on methadone, but also for diminishing the repression of drug users (including decriminalisation of possession of small amounts). Underlying these was the notion that drug use and addiction were adaptive phenomena that were a part of, rather than apart from, the wider society and its changing structures and values. Thus the policy, in the eyes of the DPD at least, was founded on the principle of developing responses within a framework of human rights and social inclusion rather than of repression and exclusion.

Reduction of harm for drug users

Reduction of harm for drug users was to involve mobilising society in terms of prevention; developing a wide network of services to limit harm and to facilitate survival and social integration of active users; and strengthening treatment and rehabilitation facilities for those who wanted to try to quit.

Prevention was seen in a broad sense as involving public discourse on social values, stigmatisation, marginalisation and demystification, rather than as an isolated issue restricted to the field of health education. In this context, a series of public forums were planned by the DPD in order to provide the opportunity for debate and exchange with sectors of the local community (including one held in conjunction with the banks). The policy also referred to the need to develop appropriate responses and to prevent the marginalisation of the wider population of drug users who were not addicted or whose circumstances were less problematic than those on the open scene. However, this aspect received little attention as the open scene and public order increasingly dominated the political debate.

Survival and crisis help (*Lebens- und Krisenhilfe*) was to be based on a network of crisis centres easily accessible to the drug scene, a first aid centre and mobile emergency service aimed at providing health care and reducing overdose deaths, and a range of supporting services including outreach, needle exchange, short-term accommodation, decentralised low-threshold methadone programmes (including a mobile unit), contact points and improved services geared to the needs of women, and a night-project for drug using prostitutes.

It was recognised that the city and the *Land* had a good system of counselling centres and abstinence-oriented therapeutic communities. The policy statement argued for these to be complemented by a detoxification clinic in the city, and by more extensive provision of methadone. In particular, it identified the need for more services, especially methadone, to be established in other parts of Hessen and for projects to encourage addicts to return to their home towns. The concepts of self-help and of the need to build possibilities for social integration and alternative, decentralised social networks, were seen as an integral part of the policy by the DPD.

Protection of citizens

Protection of citizens was seen in terms of reducing the nuisance and sense of insecurity arising from the open drug scene and from drug related crime and drug trafficking. Proposals for how this was to be achieved, including how the police would organise their priorities and activities, were not specified in the same detail as the health and social policy measures. This was partly because of continuing differences in perspective between the police, who were unwilling to relinquish their statutory responsibility to maintain public order and enforce the law, and others represented in the Monday policy group, who wanted to develop a policy which implied changes in the wider legal and social framework. It was clearly agreed, however, that it would be impossible to meet the goal of reducing the nuisance associated with the open drug scene without developing the network of services and alternatives described above.

Thus – and although it was only one aspect of the whole approach, it was the most controversial – it was agreed that the open drug scene would, to some extent at least, continue to exist. The intention was to reduce, in stepwise fashion, the concentration of the drug scene in the train station area, where it was considered to present an unacceptable nuisance, but to tolerate it for the time being in areas where it posed the least threat to the public while the network of services, especially methadone provision, was developed, and while effective steps to reverse the influx of addicts into Frankfurt were found. Exactly what 'toleration' meant in practice was left open to interpretation.

It was recognised that public support was essential. As well as organising the public forums mentioned above, the DPD gave an open commitment to respond rapidly and personally to questions and complaints from the public about drug related issues or incidents. Furthermore, it was recognised that the policy as a whole would not be accepted without measures that actually led to a reduction of tension and antagonism towards drug users amongst people living and working in the city. This meant that in addition to explaining the policy and expanding the network of services, two other issues had to be addressed. The first was that reducing the nuisance of the open scene in the city centre should not have the effect of redistributing it to residential communities across the city. The second was that it was necessary to find ways to discourage addicts from coming to Frankfurt, and to persuade non-Frankfurters to return home, or at least to leave.

DRUG POLICY IN PRACTICE

The implementation of this policy in practice involved intense debate and negotiation between the different parties, the DPD, police, prosecutor, NGOs, medical profession and others. There were important differences between the DPD and police, and, at first at least, between the DPD and most NGOs. The attempt to forge consensus on a policy that balanced the interests of different sections of the community was at the same time the source of tensions and contradictions within that policy.

Policing

The police saw maintaining control of the streets and enforcing the law as essential (both in the interests of public order and because of the principle of necessary enforcement in German law). They continued to police the open scene, though criticism, awareness of AIDS and the shifting emphasis in drug policy led them to modify important aspects of their methods. Thus by 1989 they had largely stopped confiscating syringes, and although they seized illegal drugs, the number of charges brought decreased. They also accepted the presence of an outreach drug-bus, including a needle exchange run by the NGO AIDS-Hilfe. However, in 1990, with more staff, the police intensified their activities, checking and registering an increasing number of addicts, and giving priority to reducing the size of the open scene at any one time or place by continually moving them on.

The DPD was critical of police action, which it saw as denying human rights, exacerbating the marginalisation and deterioration of addicts, and reducing the possibilities for contact with health and social services. In particular, they criticised the police for 'junkie jogging', which had intensified in 1990. They wanted to reduce the negative consequences of repression, and to foster an approach giving priority to reaching addicts, facilitating survival, reducing risk behaviours, improving health, and, in the longer term, to enabling social integration and reduced stigmatisation of drug users. In this context, tolerating the scene in a place where it would cause least nuisance was seen, not as a desirable goal in itself, but as an interim though necessary step towards changing the nature and balance of the city's response to what appeared to be a growing and intractable problem. To achieve this, however, the DPD also depended on the police to 'manage' or regulate the open scene, albeit in a different manner than before.

Crisis and survival

One key element of the policy was a network of three crisis centres to provide easily accessible contact points, street-corner cafes, washing facilities, round-the-clock crisis and emergency help, outreach, needle exchange, overnight facilities and temporary accommodation, medical help, and methadone, as well as opportunities for counselling and referral. The NGOs recognised the need for a range of harm reduction strategies, but except for one of the smaller NGOs that had been set up as an outreach and harm reduction project (AIDS-Hilfe) they did not think that they should be the ones to provide it and at first resisted changes to their counselling and social work role. Conflicts that arose included opposition to changes in working hours (many of the staff were accustomed to regular office hours); issues of professionalism (they felt they were trained to provide counselling, not to run cafes); doubts about accepting continued drug use (e.g. through needle exchanges or methadone provision) rather than treating it; and insistence on keeping their independence rather than be seen as an instrument of a policy developed by the city administration. In some cases, cooperation was also hindered by political and personal conflicts.

In most NGOs, there was a shift in the balance of how they worked, especially in providing street-corner cafes and related services, but the rate of change was slower, and the range of services more limited, than was foreseen when the strategy was first drawn up. In particular, there were problems in establishing outreach and medical crisis interventions, in developing services outside normal office hours, and in providing the accommodation and social services required for methadone provision.

The DPD dealt with this situation by diverting their funding to an NGO which was closely linked to the DPD and Department of Health, and by setting up new projects under other NGOs that were not formerly involved in the drugs field. The range of projects included a treatment centre and accommodation facilities for women, a night bus for prostitutes, accommodation for homeless addicts, and proposals for methadone programmes. Although some pilot projects had started in 1991, it was not until 1992 that these were established, and then on a relatively modest scale compared to the number of addicts in Frankfurt.

Methadone

A second key element in the strategy was the development of methadone programmes. It should be noted that the law did not allow methadone to be prescribed in the treatment of addiction, and that the attitude of the medical establishment was still negative towards such an approach. A very restricted scientific research programme of prescribing L-Polamidon to fifty HIV-positive drug using prostitutes had been proposed in 1988 by the previous CDU administration, agreed by the *Land*, and opened at the city Health Office in 1989. However, this was a public health measure based on epidemic prevention regulations which included various compulsory elements and which offered no basis for developing programmes that would be either relevant or attractive to the wider population of addicts.

Despite recommendations by the city council to extend the indications for methadone and to expand the provision of methadone, progress was delayed by conservative medical attitudes and by the cautious reactions of the insurance companies. The revised guidelines eventually agreed by a Federal Commission of doctors and insurance companies in 1991 were narrow (pregnancy, AIDS, severe illness) and the procedures, requiring a decision on each individual case by a commission at *Land* level, were cumbersome. It was also a requirement that methadone could only be provided if clients had somewhere to live and if counselling and social work help were provided. Thus it was not until 1992 that methadone treatment started to grow in Frankfurt, and only in 1993 and 1994, once the guidelines had been further revised and broadened, that the numbers expanded substantially.

Reducing the 'pull' effect of the city

A third key element was to reduce the number of addicts from outside Frankfurt. One strategy that was tried by the police was to send addicts back to their home towns, or sometimes just to transport them to the city boundary. Other tactics included withdrawing driving licences and notifying families and local authorities. None of these measures succeeded, however, since there were no services in most towns, addicts were not welcome there, and in any case the heroin market was centred in Frankfurt.

An alternative strategy adopted by the police and by the city council and DPD was to put pressure on other towns and cities to take responsibility for their own addicts and to develop services. The election of a Green/SPD government in Hessen in 1991 made discussions on drug policy easier at the level of the *Land*, and led to the development of methadone provision outside Frankfurt. It did not, however, make local authorities more eager to develop local services, nor did it have much impact on other *Länder* with more conservative policies.

Subsequently, in 1992, political and financial considerations led to restrictions on funding non-residents. Access to services such as methadone or accommodation, and social services provided by the city, was limited to addicts who had a 'passport' confirming that they were residents of Frankfurt, or who had confirmation that other local authorities would agree to pay (though this latter option raised problems, since after twelve months clients supported by other authorities qualified as Frankfurt residents and the city then became responsible for them). This was intended to reduce the 'pull' effect of the city, though it had no effect on addicts who were attracted by the easier availability and lower price of heroin.

Developments in the open drug scene

During 1991, the police reduced the level of intervention within the open scene in the Taunusanlage, though they continued to monitor it and to launch periodic raids, and they remained active in other parts of the inner city such as the train station area. The concentration of the scene in the park increased, and especially over the summer was large and active day and night, though it diminished to some extent during the winter, with a concomitant increase in the train station. A growing majority of those involved continued to be from outside Frankfurt, many of them relatively long-term intravenous heroin addicts rather than recent initiates. Research carried out in the autumn suggested a prevalence of HIV of about 20 per cent (Vogt, 1992). Problems of homelessness and poor health became increasingly urgent. The number of deaths rose to almost 150 in 1991, a high number for a relatively small city and one which caused alarm and despondency amongst those working in the field and prompted efforts to set up an outreach team and to accelerate the development of services.

Although the number of deaths dropped a little in 1992, the open scene in the Taunusanlage expanded even more as summer returned. The number of addicts registered for the first time by the police remained the same, but the proportion of non-Germans and of Germans from outside Frankfurt continued to increase. At the same time, despite the attempts of the city and railway police, illegal drug activity around the station continued, probably due, as noted above, to the geographical location of the station and to the characteristics of the space. At one point in 1991 there was a proposal, supported by the railway authorities, to reduce the visibility of the scene by erecting a large tent on an out-of-the-way site behind the station. Discussions about reducing and eventually closing the open scene gathered momentum during 1992. There were several reasons for this.

There had been many complaints about nuisance, initially from shops and businesses in the train station area, and subsequently, as the scene in the park expanded, from employees working in the banks surrounding the Taunusanlage. There was some growth in criminality related to the scene, for example street robbery, and within the scene itself there was an increase in violence and exploitation. Even though drug related crime remained relatively uncommon compared to many cities, it nonetheless aroused public anxiety in a city accustomed to a low level of street crime. At the same time, the city's drug policy, and especially the public pronouncements of the councillor responsible at political level, had attracted international attention to the situation in the city.

These circumstances coincided with the prospect of local elections early in 1993. The CDU opposition, taking advantage of public concern, started to make drug policy a political issue from late 1991. The underlying theme of the image of Frankfurt as an international centre and potential seat of the European bank probably also played a role. Over the course of 1992, public order became a very high priority in terms of political survival for the SPD/Green alliance, leading to conflicts between the SPD (who favoured closure of the park and increased enforcement) and the Green party (who felt that the policy had not yet been given a chance to work).

The closure of the park

In August 1992, the mayor (SPD) announced that the park was to be closed, though this was not implemented until the end of the year. The police were opposed to the closure until sufficient alternatives were in place, since they did not want to return to the situation where they were primarily responsible for solving the problem (though the availability in April 1992 of a hundred more police meant that they now had sufficient resources to close it if required). Most of the NGOs, who three years earlier had resisted the new drug policy, were also by now opposed to closing the park, since they feared adverse consequences, both for their clients and for the nature of their role.

Also in the summer of 1992, there was a demonstration by addicts demanding that promises about adequate services (especially methadone provision) be met. Pressure on the DPD to offer solutions increased.

Several responses were pushed through. In the summer of 1992 the number of methadone slots was expanded to 200, and the city rented a hotel to provide accommodation for 120 addicts in support of this expansion. In the autumn, Schielestrasse, a facility with accommodation for seventy addicts and a day centre for larger numbers was set up, together with a nearby methadone programme, in an old industrial area on the outskirts of the city. Plans were made for further expanding methadone provision in the following year.

The establishment of these services, in addition to the crisis centres and other projects that were being developed, was seen by the police and the Mayor as meeting the goal of providing alternatives to the open drug scene. In November 1992, the park was closed. From December onwards, the police returned to their previous practice of continually moving addicts on, and would not tolerate groups of more than three or four together within the inner city. Some, especially non-residents of Frankfurt, were expelled from the inner city, others were taken to the crisis centres where a shuttle bus transported them to Schielestrasse. However, since Schielestrasse was not widely accepted, and since in any case it could not meet the demand, many addicts returned to the station area.

Consequences of closing the park

There were several consequences of the closure of the park, taken in conjunction with the other developments described above. One, as intended, was a significant reduction in the size and visibility of the open drug scene. In particular, the Taunusanlage, after closure and renovation, remained almost entirely free of addicts. Around the station and in the nearby streets, however, there remained a circulating population of addicts, making contacts and buying and injecting drugs as hurriedly as possible before being moved on by the police.

Another consequence was a change in role and an increase in conflicts for the crisis centres. The number of clients rose, either because they were brought by the police, or because they sought refuge from the streets. The result was not only that the centres found it difficult to cope with the increased demand, but that activities which previously had taken place largely in the open scene tended to move indoors. The centres were faced with a growing problem of being used as places where contacts could be made, deals arranged, and drugs injected. These changes put the staff in the uneasy position of offering refuge and support, whilst at the same time 'policing' their clients. Some centres were overwhelmed and at times were confronted with violence.

The issue of allowing injecting to take place in the centres was particularly controversial, since the police insisted that this was illegal, whilst some centres argued that in the interests of health and reduced risk of unsafe injecting, it was better that addicts injected in more hygienic and less stressful circumstances, rather than on the street where they were continually trying to avoid the police. Some centres, including Schielestrasse, did provide facilities for injecting on the premises, which brought them into conflict with the police and prosecutor. Recently (1995) it was accepted by the public prosecutor that supervised 'fixing rooms' could operate legally, provided that only 'old', well-known addicts were admitted, that there was no dealing and that everyone brought their own drugs.

Another consequence of closing the park and increasing police pressure, of making it harder for non-Frankfurters to obtain services, and of opening methadone centres in other parts of the Hessen, was a reduction in the number of addicts from outside Frankfurt. It also led to the emergence of small open drug scenes in other cities. Despite protests from other cities, this encouraged the development of local services, at least in some areas. A broader view is that the change in police policy in Frankfurt did not reduce the problem in terms of the overall extent of addiction, but redistributed it.

But whilst the open drug scene diminished, this was probably counter-balanced by a growth in more private drug use, by a more scattered and hidden drug market that would be harder to monitor and control, and perhaps by a diversification in the substances used and injected.

Although the concentration of addicts was significantly diluted, increased police intervention against street addicts and public drug use was at odds with other aspects of a policy which aimed to reduce stigmatisation, marginal-isation and risky health behaviour. Addicts remained visible, albeit in smaller, continually mobile and furtive groups. The atmosphere surrounding this more confrontational atmosphere may well have increased the sense of rejection by people living and working in Frankfurt, even if the public order problem of large gatherings of addicts had been in part resolved.

A further dimension was that risk reduction interventions such as outreach, needle exchange and health education became more difficult to carry out, while the circumstances favouring more risky behaviour increased. This coincided with an increase in the availability and use of cocaine amongst heroin injectors (which meant a sharp increase in the frequency of injection by those who used both drugs).

Although the closure of the park dominated debate and had major repercussions on other aspects of drug policy, it should not be seen as an abandonment of important principles that were established through the multi-agency group. Thus services continued to develop and adapt. For example, one response to the changes in behaviour patterns following closure of the park was to establish nightly outreach work, including mobile needle exchange, in the streets around the station. Other examples were the expansion of methadone provision, so that by 1995 over 1,000 places were available, and a project for drug users with children.

However, the decision to close the park in 1992 was taken for political reasons and because there were, for the first time, sufficient police to make it feasible, rather than because adequate services or sufficient alternatives were really ready and in place by that time. The tension between the different objectives of policy and the interests of different sectors made it difficult to orchestrate the balance between the needs and public health interests of drug users, the right to protection of the wider society, and the political demands of the moment.

CONCLUSIONS AND IMPLICATIONS

It is difficult to assess the balance of achievements since 1988. It should be remembered that it was a growing recognition of the inadequacy of an approach that had relied heavily on repression and drug-free treatment, together with rising death rates and the emergence of HIV and AIDS, that forced a change in policy in the second half of the 1980s. And it was the increasing level of addiction in many parts of Germany, combined with the 'push' from smaller towns and more repressive regions and the 'pull' of Frankfurt as a regional and international centre, that led to a rising number of marginalised addicts who had nowhere to live and nowhere else to go. The preoccupation of local politicians and others with the open drug scene, and the obsession of the wider audience outside Frankfurt with high-profile statements, for example about decriminalisation and legalisation, combined to obscure the more down-to-earth reality of implementing changes that were clearly needed to deal with the situation that had evolved. The nature of public discourse on these controversial issues had the further effect of hiding many real achievements and valuable lessons.

Multi-agency cooperation

The regular Monday policy meetings of the key departments and the DPD played a central role in developing a workable consensus around drug policy and what was to be done. As noted above, there were at first large differences between the newly elected Green/SPD city government with its Drug Policy Division, and the police and prosecutor and others. In the subsequent evolution of the policy, the DPD came to accept that without a visible decrease in public nuisance the policy would not get public acceptance, and thus it adapted to policies that would fit the goals of public order. Conversely, the police recognised that it was not their job to be dealing with people who were sick, that repression of users was not the primary solution, and that alternatives in the field of health and social policy were crucial. The Public Prosecutor, NGOs and other parties also changed some of their positions over time.

This process of forging consensus was not without its difficulties. For example, the police tended to see health and social service interventions in terms of social order measures, and the role of policing in terms of pressuring addicts to go to the services (as well as chasing dealers). This was a point of ideological conflict with some NGOs, who saw the siting of Schielestrasse as collaborating with the authorities to 'cleanse' the city by shifting social problems out of the sight of society and into a peripheral part of the city. Similar criticisms were voiced over the setting up of a night bus for drug using prostitutes near the motorway area to which the police had moved them from a middle-class inner-city residential area.

There were also, at times, differences in interpretation between senior managers who took part in policy discussions, and their staff who were involved at the operational level. Thus the police responsible for street-level work and the social workers in the crisis centres sometimes had different views on the situation than their superiors, and also tended to have different levels of conflict with each other. The Friday meetings of NGOs, police and the DPD concerning practical issues were of great value in improving understanding at this level. These meetings also gave a valuable opportunity to exchange information about current trends and what was happening in the drug scene (though not information that might have compromised individuals).

Despite differences in underlying perspectives, the persistence and commitment by almost all parties involved in the city to maintain a coordinated approach, notably through the regular Monday meetings, should be seen as a notable achievement and endorsement of the value of such an approach. In many cases, it proved possible to compromise in the practice without giving up important underlying principles, even though this did not resolve all the contradictions that inevitably resulted.

The lesson is that to set up a multi-agency forum is not enough. It is also essential to involve senior managers from the respective agencies so that there is a direct link to policy decisions, as well as to provide a parallel forum where those involved at the operational level can learn to work together and share perceptions of the situation. Further, it is vital to establish a clear structure and programme of work that allows cooperation to be maintained and carried forward. In this regard, the value of a full-time secretariat (the DPD, consisting of six people) linked to the policy process must be strongly underlined.

Harm reduction, public order and the police

There were several important ways in which the police modified their actions to take account of the need to reduce the risks of HIV transmission. Initially, they stopped confiscating syringes and cooperated with outreach workers and needle exchanges. They also reduced the extent to which they arrested drug users (though they did not stop confiscating drugs and registering users). Subsequently they firmly supported the development of services and the expansion of methadone provision. By 1994, there was even some support for controlled distribution of heroin. They were also in favour of supervised facilities for 'safe' injecting, though they could not officially permit these until the Public Prosecutor provided the legal basis.

Whilst important and concrete progress was made in terms of cooperation between health and social services and the police regarding issues of public health, it was also clear that there were limits. The police were not willing to relinquish their role in maintaining public order and controlling the streets, and insisted on their right to intervene when they considered that it was necessary. Despite these limits, they did not close the park until they felt that alternative services were available. When they did take action, they did not do so unannounced, but only after many months of discussion with other parties.

There is no doubt that active participation in the policy group played an important part in the changes in police practice. The international context, including visits to cities such as Amsterdam and Zürich, was also influential. One conclusion is that law enforcement policies and practices have a major impact not only on the drug scene but also on the role and activities of other agencies. There is sometimes a tendency for NGOs or health authorities to overlook the police when developing risk reduction strategies and interventions, or to see them merely as an inconvenient force which keep arresting their clients.

The lesson here is that it is important for health authorities, NGOs, outreach teams and others to take the public order perspective seriously as a key dimension of the environment in which they work, and to involve the police in a meaningful way in policy discussion (United Nations, 1995). This of course depends on the willingness of the police to see the value of such participation.

Cooperation between NGOs and local authorities

In some cases, community interventions evolve through NGOs or self-help groups, in other cases they are implemented by local health or social service authorities. The perspectives from which they approach community intervention differ. Many NGOs develop out of concern for the well-being of specific groups, and tend to act as advocates in the interests of those groups. Local authorities, whilst not lacking in concern, often act from the point of view of public health or protection of the wider community, and are more accountable (and influenced by) public opinion and political exigencies. They also often operate within a more hierarchical and bureaucratic structure. In contrast, NGOs tend to adopt a more democratic form of organisation and to pride themselves on their independence of official strictures.

Some of these factors were present in Frankfurt. The DPD needed the cooperation of the NGOs in changing the emphasis of health and social policy from counselling and therapy towards harm reduction and crisis intervention. As noted earlier, most NGOs resisted change and were reluctant to be coordinated by the DPD. The response of the DPD was a mixture of increased efforts at consultation and the use of funding, mainly via other NGOs, to alter the direction of future service development. The regular Friday meetings were originally set up to facilitate cooperation between the DPD and NGOs and, just as important, between the different NGOs. Subsequently this became a broader forum for discussing practical cooperation and exchanging experiences and information on current developments in the drug scene.

Although the background to setting up the DPD included various political and personal tensions, the DPD staff responsible for service development and involved in many of the negotiations about new projects was widely liked and accepted by them. This was important in maintaining links, developing a degree of trust and goodwill, and encouraging change.

The lesson to be learned is that establishing a multi-agency policy is not sufficient. If partnership with non-governmental and other organisations is to bear fruit, then real recognition of their differences with official structures is essential, and time and opportunities for regular discussion must be made available. The characteristics of the people responsible for this liaison are one key to successful communication and cooperation. This latter point, of course, also applies to liaison with other organisations such as the police or the medical profession.

Assessing needs, evaluating results

The coordination group and the creation of the DPD not only arose in response to visible needs that demanded better solutions, but in turn provided a framework within which to assess and at times redefine those needs. Some needs, for example for outreach, crisis help, health care and accommodation, were readily apparent in general terms, but required clarification in order to ensure that interventions were appropriate. Other needs were less obvious and rather ill-defined.

Some of this needs assessment was done through critical appraisal and discussion of existing information. Some was done through research, for example a study carried out in the open drug scene in the autumn of 1991 (Vogt, 1992). Another example was a working group set up in 1990 to examine the needs of women drug users. This identified a range of needs and led to a range of practical interventions concerning accommodation, counselling, treatment and health care options geared to specific needs regarding AIDS, children, violence, prostitution and employment.

However, the emphasis on the open drug scene meant that other aspects were neglected. For example, there was no research, and very little knowledge, about drug use in the city as a whole, nor about the prevalence, problems and needs of regular drug users who were not involved in the open scene. Whilst some data were collected, for example on drug deaths or users registered by the police, few data were collected in a systematic fashion in order to monitor trends or evaluate the impact of different aspects of policy.

Developing a policy, and defending it, are strengthened if systematic information is collected in order to clarify needs and evaluate both process and outcomes. It would have been useful (though unusual!) if an independent evaluation had been considered at an early stage.

Public relations and public debate

The importance of public opinion and of key community groups such as businesses, shops, banks and residents was recognised by all involved. Three public forums were held (one in the train station, one with the banks, and a third on cocaine) though it was not clear what effect these had, and two further planned events were not held. Another strategy, mentioned above, was to make the DPD responsive to questions and complaints from the public, though at times the volume of work almost paralysed them.

The most valuable approach was probably the cooperation that was established between the agencies involved in the Monday group regarding the presentation of drug policy and policy developments to the media, especially the local media. This did not of course prevent the media, politicians or others from putting their own gloss on what was taking place in the city, but it did mean that there was a coherence in how decisions and differences were presented, and that the level of debate was more informed.

'Push' and 'pull' factors

Many cities face the problem of being attractive to drug users, addicts and suppliers from surrounding regions and even from further afield, especially if they are major centres of economic activity and trade, leisure and associated services, transport and communications. At one level, this may be an inevitable correlate of the wider role that cities play as centres for the exchange of goods and services of all kinds. At another level it can create serious difficulties, especially if the (visible) concentration of a phenomenon such as drug addiction rises above an acceptable level.

The 'push' factors that may encourage addicts to leave their home towns include stigmatisation, rejection and repressive policies, difficulties in obtaining supplies of drugs, or a lack of services and other alternatives. 'Pull' factors may include the greater anonymity offered by a city and the possibilities of finding a supportive subculture, a larger drug market with (usually) lower prices, and the perception of a wider range of opportunities for generating income. If policies are less intolerant or if there is a greater range of attractive services (e.g. methadone provision), then this too is likely to be a 'pull' factor.

In Frankfurt the 'push' factors were somewhat reduced by the development of drug scenes and drug markets in other cities following the closure of the open scene, and by the development there of services, especially methadone provision. This may have been associated with some changes in repressive attitudes and tolerance, but this is hard to assess.

The 'pull' factors were also somewhat reduced by the closure of the open scene and by police pressure (especially on non-Frankfurters) and perhaps also by restricting methadone and some other services to Frankfurt residents. Although the closure of the open scene may have made it a little more difficult for strangers to obtain drugs, and shifted some of the distribution to other cities, heroin, cocaine and other drugs almost certainly remained more easily available and cheaper in relation to smaller towns. At the same time, as noted above, there were other consequences of closing the open scene which had some negative effects for services and drug users from the city.

The lesson from the experience of Frankfurt is that it is not possible to reduce the attraction effect of a city solely by attempts to expel addicts and force them to return home. It is also essential that alternatives are pursued by other municipalities and regions. This in turn raises issues concerning the wider environment within which the policy of any individual city has to operate, including national legislation, government policy, methadone regulations, insurance company policies, and the relation of the city to the region. These are not the focus of this chapter, but it is clear that they have an important role in determining what is possible and how. The emergence of city networks reflects the concerns that many of them share (Frankfurt am Main, 1991).

Stigma, inclusion or exclusion?

One of the main concepts on which the new policy was based, at least from the point of view of the DPD and some of its partners, was that it was necessary to reduce the stigmatisation and rejection of drug users and drug addicts.

Although there was a reduction in the level of repression directed towards drug users, and a concommitant increase in provision (and funding) for healthcare, social services and housing, there was not much evidence of increased acceptance of drug addicts by the community as a whole. Despite objections from some NGOs and others to policies that moved addicts out of sight, the overall thrust of policy reflected a historical tradition of regulating social problems in a way that was a microcosm of how society is regulated in terms of space, residence, work and leisure. In this, the development of drug policy paralleled that towards prostitution. The city regulated where and how sex workers operated by using long-existing 'zoning laws' to limit prostitution to a few specific buildings in the station area and to establish zones where it was permitted, away from commercial or residential areas and near industrial sites or motorways.

One lesson may be that attempts to reduce stigmatisation and exclusion, and to bring addicts fully into the circle of 'normal' society, are limited within the constraints of existing social structures. This is but one example of the problem of achieving equal rights and treatment for unpopular minorities. In this case, it is particularly hard to explain what 'cleansing' means to the majority and what it can mean for the minority. At the very least, improving the acceptance of addicts while not condoning addiction is likely to be a much longer process than could be expected in the time-scale covered in the present case.

Another lesson, especially if stigmatisation remains a reality, is that there is a need for a clear ethical perspective on the rights of unpopular minorities, such as addicts, to human dignity, equal treatment, and access to services. Without this, there are real dangers of sliding towards ever more repressive and symbolic acts of exclusion, with the likelihood of ever-increasing negative consequences, not only for the individuals involved, but also for the wider communities of which they are still a part.

Ideology, pragmatism and policy

The original formulation of drug policy at the time of the election of the Green/SPD city government and the setting up of the DPD was based on strong ideological commitments to an alternative approach. The political statements that were made, and still are, for example around the Frankfurt Resolution which was passed in 1990, have sometimes been discussed at a somewhat rarefied level in terms of 'encouraging' versus 'fighting' drugs and drug addiction. However, the practice of drug policy, although fed by ideological perspectives, was driven by pragmatic concerns arising both from political expediency and from the concrete day-to-day realities of serious social problems concerning public health and public safety.

From this point of view, the practice of drug policy was not about 'encouraging' or 'condoning' drugs and drug addiction, but about how best to manage a situation where benefits in terms of one objective were likely to be at the expense of negative consequences in terms of another. No one in Frankfurt, regardless of their stance on drug policy, thought that drug injecting or the open drug scene was a 'good thing'. Rather, the issue was how to find an acceptable approach that was more constructive than that which almost all involved agreed had not been working in the past, an approach that would reduce the health and social costs to individuals and to society, and at the same time respect the human rights and dignity of drug users as members of that same society.

Endnote: public health and public safety

So did the policy work? This is not an easy question, since the complex range of factors is difficult to untangle, and crucial evidence has still to be obtained and analysed in depth. However, some observations are possible.

The policy succeeded in redressing the imbalance between repression and health and social measures, and in improving the delivery and uptake of services, especially those that aimed to reduce adverse health and social consequences for drug addicts. It is hard to measure accurately the impact that this had on the health of addicts in general, though there are some pointers. The number of deaths fell sharply from 147 in 1991 and 127 in 1992, to 68 in 1993 and 60 in 1994, though it is not clear how far this was a result of reductions in risky drug using behaviour as opposed to a reduction in the number of addicts coming into Frankfurt. It is also difficult to evaluate precisely the effect on the spread of HIV, since reliable data are not available on annual incidence (seroconversion) rates. However, the prevalence of HIV amongst drug injectors in Frankfurt was estimated to be 15–20 per cent in 1993, suggesting no increase since 1991. Amongst addicts who died in Frankfurt, the proportion who were HIV positive decreased from 30 per cent in 1987 to 11–13 per cent between 1991 and 1993.

In terms of public order, the open scene was reduced and public anxiety allayed to some extent, though this had some negative consequences for the crisis centres, and possibly also for the risk behaviours of addicts. It is not clear whether the overall level of drug related crime in the city fell, but crime associated with a large concentration of addicts probably did. In the longer term, the policy may not have affected prevalence, but rather increased the proportion of drug users and of the drug market that is hidden. The aspect of the policy concerned with reducing the 'pull' effect of the city also contributed to an increased visibility of drug users in other parts of the *Land*.

The policy appears to have been less successful in reducing the stigmatisation and marginalisation of addicts as a category, though at the individual level there were many addicts who benefited. Changes in stereotypes of addiction cannot be expected within a short time frame, and the possibilities in the longer term may be limited. Every society 'needs' its outsiders, and their relationship with society is likely to remain ambivalent at best. The question is how to respond to those outsiders in ways that are humane, that minimise the damage that arises both for them and for the society, and that maximise the number of individuals who benefit.

ACKNOWLEDGEMENTS

Many thanks to the people who gave their time to talk about the situation in Frankfurt: Wolfgang Barth, Herbert Drexler, Peter Frerichs, Volker Happel, Martina Hetzel, Cora Molloy, Peter Noller, Roswitha Prinz, Petra Schnatz, Werner Schneider, Urban Weber.

REFERENCES

Deutscher Bundestag (ed.) (1988) *AIDS: Fakten und Konsequenzen. Zwischenbericht der Enquête-Kommission 'Gefahren von AIDS und wirksame Wege zu ihrer Eindämmung' des Deutschen Bundetages* [AIDS: Facts and Consequences. Interim Report of the Commission of Enquiry 'Effective Ways of Reducing the Risks of AIDS'], Bonn: Deutscher Bundestag.

Frankfurt am Main (1991a) *Documentation of the 1st Conference: European Cities at the Centre of the Illegal Trade in Drugs*, Frankfurt am Main: Drug Policy Division.

—— (1991a) *Mit Drogenabhängigen Leben! Rahmenplan zur Gestaltung der Drogenpolitik in Frankfurt am Main* [To Live with Drug Addicts!], Frankfurt am Main: Drug Policy Division.

Kindermann, W., Sickinger, R., Hedrich, D. and Kindermann, S. (1989) *Drogenabhängig: Lebenswelten zwischen Szene, Justiz, Therapie und Drogenfreiheit* [Drug Addicted: Life between the Drug Scene, Justice, Therapy and Abstinence], Freiburg: Lambertus-Verlag.

Noller, P. (1991) 'Mythos Heroin: Szene und Politik in Frankfurt am Main' [Heroin Myths: Scene and Policy in Frankfurt], in F.O. Brauerhoch (ed.) *Frankfurt am Main, Stadt, Soziologie und Kultur*, Frankfurt am Main: Verlag Vervuert.

Schneider, W. and Happel, H. V. (1987) *Ausstieg aus der Drogenabhängigkeit am Beispiel der Selbstheiler* [How to Quit Drugs: the Example of Self-recovery], Zwischenbericht des Forschungsprojekts 'Selbstheiler', Wiesbaden: Hessiches Ministerium für Arbeit und Soziales.

United Nations (1995) *Reduction of Illicit Demand for Drugs: Prevention Strategies including Community Participation*, Report of the Secretariat, Economic and Social Council, E/CN.7/1995/5, Vienna: United Nations Economic and Social Council.

Vogt, I. (1992) *Offene Szene in Frankfurt am Main: Abschlussbericht* [The Open Drug Scene in Frankfurt: Final Report], Frankfurt am Main: Drug Policy Division.

Chapter 5

'"E" types and dance divas'
Gender research and community prevention

Sheila Henderson

The use of illegal drugs among young people is currently cause for public concern in Britain. Since the late 1980s, empirical evidence points to the fact that the extent and variety of drug use has increased (Balding, 1994; ISDD, 1994; Parker *et al.*, 1995). Recent evidence also suggests that young women are involved as much as, and in the case of some drugs, more than, young men (Measham *et al.*, 1993). Placed alongside other 'youth' statistics in the public mind, such as 'joyriding', this phenomenon has been perceived as a social threat, debatably supplanting HIV/AIDS in magnitude.

While young people's sexuality and, more generally, injecting use of drugs have received research and policy attention, the relationship between non-injecting drug use and sexual behaviour among young people has received far less (Ford, 1990). Much drug taking among young people takes places in leisure settings. It is perceived as normal and an integral part of a popular youth culture. It is therefore very different from the problem of injecting which has formed the major focus of research.

Studies of young people's sexuality have demonstrated the important role played by gender in the social acquisition of male and female sexuality and in the negotiation of sexual encounters (Holland *et al.*, 1992, 1993; Wight, 1993). These accounts have highlighted the constraints upon female sexual options and choices but have rarely been grounded in the specific sexual cultures that frame them. While the role of gender in the use of drugs has received some recent attention, this has rarely been in the context of youth culture.

The role of research in HIV prevention has been varied. Community-based HIV prevention initiatives which employ ethnographic research methods, often in combination with outreach techniques and an emphasis on including the 'researched' in the research process, have been a particularly notable example of the practical application of research (see Chapters 9 and 12). However, like much research on illicit drug use and risk taking in the post-AIDS era, the focus of such initiatives has been largely on 'hard to reach' populations whose behaviours are perceived to put them most at risk of HIV. Young recreational drug users are often 'easy to reach' in the sense that they can often be found using drugs in large numbers in public leisure settings. They therefore require a somewhat different community-based approach than previously adopted.

Drawing on the Young Sexuality and Recreational Drug Use Project, which was conducted in Manchester between October 1991 and October 1993 (see also Henderson, 1993a, 1993b, 1993c, 1993d, 1994a, 1994b), this chapter aims to examine the relationship between drug use, sexuality and sexual risk taking among young women who used drugs recreationally within the specific setting of the club or 'rave' scene. It begins with a brief introduction to the 'dance drug' phenomenon and the research project, and moves on to contrast findings on gender, drug use, sexuality in general and in the context of 'dance drug' use, with existing research perspectives. The practical implications for HIV prevention are also discussed.

THE 'DANCE DRUG' PHENOMENON

The use of Ecstasy (MDMA) among a small group of people in the fashion, media and music industries in Britain was reported in 1985 (Nasmyth, 1985). Seizures of the drug by police steadily increased from this time and 1987 saw the first evidence that MDMA was being manufactured in Britain and the first widespread use of the drug in major cities (Redhead, 1993). Mainstream media coverage of the 'Evil of Ecstasy' made its public debut in 1988 (*Sun*, 1988). The context of its use was at the root of public concern: the illicit nature of its use, the nuisance value and the potentially subversive element with large numbers of young people gathering together to dance all night to 'house' music under the influence of stimulant and psychedelic drugs in warehouses, fields and clubs. Official surveillance and legislation followed but, instead of curbing the phenomenon, the Licensing Act 1988 and the Entertainments (Increased Penalties) Act 1990 simply changed its scale and structure. In legal club venues as well as the more usual illicit venues, what came to be known as the 'rave' scene thrived. The effects of Ecstasy, dubbed the 'hug' or 'love' drug, had been central to defining the initial culture. A general feeling of well-being, confidence, heightened sensations, love towards one's fellow human beings and the ability to dance energetically played an important role not only in determining the kind of social interaction associated with this phenomenon but also in making it an attractive leisure option. Widespread media coverage, although alarmist, made a considerable contribution to the phenomenon's high profile. Popular youth culture – from nightclubs and fashion retail outlets to youth TV, style magazines and even the football terraces – was flooded and 'rave' became big business (*Smash Hits*, 1992).

Despite perennial warnings of its 'short-lived phase' nature, the summer of 1993 saw little sign of decline in what was now the 'dance drug' phenomenon, despite increased official surveillance of its more subcultural elements and proposed new legal curbs. The music, the dress styles, the associated cultures and the groups of young people involved diversified as the popularisation process continued. More powerful psychedelic drugs, barbiturates and rock cocaine also entered the drug 'menu'.

RESEARCH ON YOUNG WOMEN, SEXUALITY AND RECREATIONAL DRUG USE

This project was conducted between October 1991 and October 1993 by the author in association with the Lifeline (Drug) Project, Manchester. Funded by the North West Regional Health Authority, it focused specifically on the use of 'dance drugs' among young women 15–25 years of age, with a view to delivering an account of young women's participation within the 'dance drug' culture. It also set out to describe the young women's sexual and social lifestyles so as to provide a 'market research' basis for the development of appropriate HIV/AIDS and risk reduction intervention strategies.

In all, 304 young women and 70 young men participated in the project. The findings reported here are drawn from the main study which comprised thirty in-depth individual interviews with young women accompanied by a lifestyle questionnaire. A broadly representative sample was recruited via 'snowballing' from contacts made through social networking, the Lifeline project, flyers placed in bars, cafes, clubs, clothes and record shops, an advertisement placed in a local women's magazine and, in a minority of cases, drug agency clients.

The young women interviewed were from a range of backgrounds and occupations and were between 15 and 25 years of age (mean age 21 years). All were involved in the north-west club 'scene', and over half had been involved for two or more years. Two young women had been into the 'scene' but had never experimented with drugs other than cannabis (which they had rejected after one or two attempts), and one had tried Ecstasy and amphetamine only once (she had also experimented with cannabis on rare occasions). The remainder had been through periods of weekly use of (varying combinations of) Ecstasy, amphetamine and LSD ranging from three months' to three years' duration. Eight young women had stopped taking drugs other than cannabis entirely at the time of interview and seven had reduced the frequency of their drug use.

Twenty-two young women had experimented with cannabis prior to involvement in the 'dance scene'. The 'dance drug' culture was not, therefore, a major factor in recruiting these young women to illegal drug use *per se* but its role in introducing them to the use of Class A illegal drugs and amphetamine sulphate should not be understated – twenty-three young women first used such drugs in this context. Drug use was, like the music, dancing and social interaction, an important component of the culture for all the young women except two – whose initial lack of interest in or even disdain for the culture was clearly stated, making drug use the only attraction in becoming involved.

GENDER AND DRUG USE

The literature on illicit drug use has a number of limitations regarding the issue of gender. All too often studies have ignored it as an explicit influential factor, with the result that, by default, the male experience has been presented as a general one. Although sharpened by AIDS reporting, coverage of women's drug use more generally has been notable for its designation of those involved as deviant, marginal and morally culpable (Henderson, 1994a). The most familiar recent example of this introduced the phenomenon of 'crack babies'. The moral attitudes, if not the sensationalism, concerning women's drug use identifiable in the media are reflected to some degree in the literature on women and drugs. Early contributions to a drugs literature dominated by medical and psychological explanations of drug use, when considering women at all, cast women's drug use as a deviation from 'normal' femininity and explained it, at best, as a compensation for physical or mental deficiencies, at worst as a disease (Rosenbaum, 1981; Cuskey, 1982). These disease and deviance models tended to focus on women's role as mothers and arose from a concern about the effects of drug use on pregnancy outcomes defined purely in relation to the baby (Blenheim Project, 1989).

Contributions to the literature from the women's health movement have been critical of the 'disease' and 'deviance' models of women's drug use, viewing women's drug dependence instead in the light of broader social forms of dependence and gender inequality. Although alcohol and tranquilliser use dominate this literature, non-prescribed illegal drugs have also featured. A key early article argued that:

> Drug dependent females are seen as characteristically pathetic, passive, psychologically and socially inadequate, isolated and incapable of shouldering responsibilities . . . . These images are drawn from a view of women's major role as centrally responsible for the 'private' side of life – housework, childcare, emotional support and family servicing . . . . The illegal addict is seen as first rejecting and then being rendered incapable of performing these functions effectively by a lifestyle which is initially wilfully perverse and then inescapably pathetic . . . . Female dependence is a reality – female drug dependence is an inappropriate and undesirable side-effect to be redirected to more convenient and controllable forms of dependence.
>
> (Perry, 1979:1)

In Britain, this early seminal work has seen little follow-up in recent years (Dorn et al.,1992; Ettorre, 1992; Henderson, 1990; Oppenheimer, 1991; Thom, 1991; Waterson and Ettorre, 1989), the volume of the literature being predominantly American and latterly Australian (Broom and Stevens, 1991; Roth, 1991; Sargent, 1991, 1992; Wodak, 1990).

Although no longer considered deviant, women who use drugs still ultimately tend to be viewed as victims – of social circumstances, men's power, or their addictive personality. Sociological research specifically focusing on women's drug use has developed little in the fourteen years since Perry's article. A study published in 1981 (Rosenbaum, 1981) was, until recently, the most notable in-depth sociological study of how injecting drug use fits into women's lives. Taylor's ethnographic study of women injectors in Glasgow (Taylor, 1993) importantly departs from existing accounts in the overall picture of female drug use it presents. Contrary to previous research findings which have highlighted women's dependence on men for acquiring and administering their drugs, their involvement in prostitution, their supposed irresponsibility, passivity, greater deviance and psychological disturbance, Taylor's account of women's drug 'careers' portrays the *active* part played by women in illicit drug use.

Findings presented here from the Young Women, Sexuality and Recreational Drug Use Project also challenge previous understandings of women's drug use, although in a different context – the recreational use of different drugs by a different population in a different setting. The young women involved were open and more than happy to talk about their drug use. They consumed drugs in public leisure settings in the pursuit of pleasure, they often acquired their own drugs, were sometimes involved in low-level dealing and were, on the whole, able to maintain a range of other life options and aspirations beyond the context of their drug use. From a wide range of backgrounds, they were very much part of a mainstream youth culture to which drugs are integral and which, while not hermetically sealed off from wider social inequalities relating to class, gender, ethnicity, sexual orientation, and even disability, nonetheless appears to hold the possibility of allowing greater social equality. This 'democratisation' of popular culture has been noted elsewhere (Redhead, 1993).

Clear gender differences were, however, obvious and just over half the sample experienced them as such. Their accounts suggested that the social expectations of young women with regard to drugs were different from those of young men. For example, young women felt themselves less likely, on the whole, to take large doses of relevant drugs (Henderson, 1993a). Other gender differences related to the physical effects of drug use. While menstrual problems were obviously related to biological difference, the commonly experienced phenomenon of weight loss was more clearly linked to socially defined gender difference. Except in extreme cases of loss of two or more stones in weight (12.5 kilos), young women viewed weight loss as an advantageous side effect of 'dance drug' use, perhaps reflecting a greater social emphasis upon physical appearance as an important part of female identity. Yet other gender differences were notable in access to the 'dance drug' culture. Young women were, for example, less likely to be searched by a venue's security staff, less likely to become one of the most powerful figures in the 'scene' – a DJ – and less likely to be involved in dealing other than at a low level. They were also more likely to be able to access drugs, transport and entrance to a venue purely on the basis of their appearance. The gender differences most pertinent to this discussion, however, are related to sexuality. Before examining these, it is helpful to contextualise the drugs/sexuality connection.

DRUGS AND SEXUALITY

The advent of HIV/AIDS has given rise to a new body of research on sexuality. The roles of sexual behaviour, perceptions of risk, sexual identity and knowledge about HIV/AIDS all continue to receive research attention. The relationship between drug use and sexual behaviour has also featured in this literature with three main areas of research focus: the disinhibitory effects of alcohol on sexual behaviour; the disinhibitory effects of cocaine on sexual behaviour, particularly in the context of prostitution; and the injecting use of illicit drugs, where the sharing of injecting equipment initially took precedence over sexual transmission of the virus as a prevention concern.

The limitations of this research on the relationship between drug taking and sexual risk behaviour were discussed in a recent and rare literature review (Rhodes and Stimson, 1994). This concluded that the determinants of the relationship between drug use and sexual behaviour (pharmacological, social, situational and cultural) remain unclear and current understanding rests as much upon common sense as on empirical evidence. It also suggested the need for research perspectives which recognise that 'individual behaviour and individual understandings of the use of drugs in relation to sexual behaviour are mediated by a complex interaction between cognition and culture' (Rhodes and Stimson, 1994:221). This is necessary in order for important distinctions to be made between 'effects' which are perceived to be pharmacological and those effects which are socially constructed in different cultures of drug use and sexual behaviour.

Existing research on the relationship between drug use and sexuality has focused predominantly upon the behaviour of injecting drug users, prostitutes and gay men. Factors constraining the practice of safer sex among injecting drug users, prostitutes and their sexual partners comprise the bulk of gender concerns within this literature (McKeganey and Barnard, 1992), but are not necessarily translatable to the drug and sexual culture in question.

The project's main study of thirty young women aimed to contribute to the literature on drug use and sexuality in a number of respects: by focusing upon the recreational and non-injecting use of drugs by a mainstream population; by examining the sexual dynamics and the role of drug use within a specific youth culture; by employing a wider definition of sexuality as a complex socially constructed field involving far more than simple biological imperatives; and by attempting to distinguish between different components of the relationship between drug use and sexuality. While rare, other studies which specifically focus on the relationship between drug use, sexuality and social context do exist (Lewis, 1991; Matthews, 1993). They do not, however, attempt to distinguish between the social, cultural and pharmacological components of the accounts they give. The following account makes as initial attempt.

THE ROLE OF PHARMACOLOGY

It is curious that a drug which can increase emotional closeness, enhance receptivity to being sexual and would be chosen as a sexual enhancer, does not increase the desire to initiate sex.

(Buffum and Moser, 1986)

This finding from a study of MDMA and, in the researchers' words, 'sexual function' would appear to lend scientific support for the now established common-sense understanding of the sexual mores of the 'dance scene' – that sexual and sensual feelings are abundant but sexual activity is rare. However, even if the role of the social setting of drug use is not considered, further qualification is required. First, current knowledge of drug markets does not facilitate any kind of accurate classification of the content of 'street' drugs. Consequently, knowledge of purity and actual dosage of a specific drug is poor and the effects described by users may not necessarily result from, in the case of Ecstasy, MDMA. In addition, little is known about the relationship between the pharmacological effects of specific drugs, the psychological preconception of those effects and the actual experience. These factors increase the already difficult task of establishing the precise role played by the pharmacological effects of specific drugs in defining the social codes of specific cultures. The following attempt to examine the relationship between drugs and sexuality is therefore a preliminary investigation.

THE 'DANCE SCENE' AS A SEXUAL CULTURE

The sexualisation of cultural components

The 'dance scene' was changing and fragmenting at the time of the study and has continued to do so. The 'scene' now comprises a wide range of nocturnal (and even daytime) events appealing to diverse populations – from main-stream city-centre nightclubs offering 'chart hits' purely for profit through to large-scale illegal events in rural settings. It is therefore difficult to general-ise. An increasing sexualisation of the culture has, however, accompanied this popularisation and fragmentation and is more obvious in some sectors than others. One of the more popular magazines associated with 'the scene' reflected this sexualisation as early as 1992 in articles such as 'Sex on Drugs' and 'Lust in New York', as well as an editorial which reflected that:

The sexual temperature is definitely rising . . . . Over in New York the clubs are heaving in the biggest explosion of lust since the backroom bacchanalia from before AIDS hit the States . . . these clubbers have been wise to AIDS since before they were having sex. But awareness of the virus doesn't seem to be stopping them.

(*Mixmag*, 1992:2)

Other components of the culture have reflected this sexualisation. Clothing, in many venues, moved on during the research period from the earlier androgyny through a range of skimpy and figure-hugging guises for both men and women, with notable borrowing from gay leather and rubber scenes. Flyers advertising venues, club nights and events also became more sexualised during the period of the research. While it would be unfair to suggest that they are totally representative of flyers in general, titles such as *Flesh*, *Love Ranch*, *Spank*, *Eden* and *Luvdup* indicate the general image of some sections of the 'scene'. There was also a growing use of sexualised images of women in this context. The use of professional dancers in sexualised outfits as an additional focus and mood orchestrator also increased in some sectors and the overall balance of the popularity of a specific type of music in the 'scene' as a whole changed during the research period from frenetic electronic sounds to more tuneful 'funky' styles.

Sexual codes within the culture

Common-sense understanding of the 'dance scene' in the UK suggests that, in contrast to other nocturnal leisure pursuits, pride of place is not given to pursuit of a sexual partner in the repertoire of potential pleasures on offer. Rather, sensations of the 'Mind, Body or Soul', a group feeling of togetherness, are the more likely motivation for participating. These key distinguishing cultural features appear to reflect the role played by Ecstasy in defining this culture, but separating out the influence of the drug from a range of other factors – such as individual preconceptions and expectations of the culture – is difficult. This is further complicated by the difficulty of distinguishing between the obvious survival of the general ethos of the culture – with its emphasis upon sensuality and togetherness – and its relationship to actual (and changing) events and experiences in a diversifying culture.

This young woman's account provides an interesting summary of the sexual codes identified within the culture during the course of the study. It also indicates both the survival of the overall ethos of the 'scene' in a popular venue in the north-west in 1993 and some contradictions that it has encouraged:

Your main objective isn't to cop off and you don't think people are looking at you all night. They probably do but it doesn't feel like that. Lads dance a lot more than they would at other clubs and it seems there's a lot more boys and girls together rather than boys at one side of the dance floor and girls in the middle of the dance floor . . . lads will come up and talk to you more . . . but often the last thing on their mind is getting off with you . . . I enjoy getting off my head and dancing and that's what I go out for. I think it's very easy to go out and meet someone, have sex. Not that I personally do but I can see why some people do. When you're all 'loved up' you want to cuddle and hold people and this could progress to sex. Also people look really nice when you're off your head but the next day it's like, 'Ugh! what an ugly bastard' . . . . When you go out raving you tend to become one of the lads and I think it takes a certain type of girl to go raving anyway. There are a lot of naive girls these days who go but it didn't start off like that. These days there's really tarty girls at the clubs and whilst it never annoys me [it's just funny] it is very different to three years ago when there was no emphasis on femininity . . . . I wouldn't like to go out with anyone who hadn't been out raving, I couldn't go out with a lad who always went down the pub and hadn't tried drugs.

(17-year-old factory worker)

All the young women in the sample reproduced the image of the culture as one in which the pursuit of sex was well down on the evening's agenda – outweighed by the attraction of going out with a crowd of friends and participating in a large group experience with a range of sensual experiences on offer. The perceived sexual codes operating within this culture were contrasted with the more customary emphasis upon sexual availability in other club scenes and found to be more favourable. This despite increasing reports of, in their words, 'shady' characters and atmospheres at raves due perhaps to a greater presence of organised crime.

This 19-year-old secretary found nightclubs to be an unsatisfactory experience before she discovered the 'dance scene':

It's like a cattlemarket, you know what I mean? Everybody goes out, goes to the bar, gets a drink, gets pissed and like the lads are all over the girls and all the girls dance around their handbags. I feel now that it's a dead narrow point of view . . . it's not really enjoying yourself . . . you end up making a fool of yourself at the end of the night . . . you're throwing up, you can't walk home, you get ripped off when you get in the taxi 'cos they see you're drunk . . . it was going nowhere for me. I don't like alcohol much anyway.

FEMALE SEXUALITY IN THE 'DANCE DRUG' CONTEXT

Sexual safety was clearly part of the scene's attraction for young women but so too were a range of sexualised experiences. While some young women described the experiences available in this context in terms of sensuality, other accounts were decidedly sexual. This 21-year-old student went so far as to describe the overall experience as 'safe sex', and other descriptions were similar:

> It's so much more fun and it's not nearly as messy ... the whole atmosphere, going to a club [is like] the nice parts of sex because you have physical contact with people and you feel dead sexy, you feel really happy. Happy about yourself and happy about other people and you are close to people that are friendly without having to worry about the other side, it's almost like safe sex. It's a shame you have to take drugs for that, that's the way it is really.

One respondent recounted an occasion on which she had been overwhelmed by the experience:

> It's more of an all-over orgasm. It's been too much before, in fact I've had to run off and go and be sick. It was just one of those nights that everything was absolutely wonderful and just dancing quite close and any physical contact, it was just getting higher and higher and higher then suddenly it's too much and I had to run off fairly quickly.
>
> (20-year-old secretary)

Such accounts tend to confirm the overall image of the culture as sensual – even sexual – but far from the simple narrative of hunting a sexual partner. They also suggest a degree of auto-eroticism in which it is difficult to isolate the contribution of the effects of Ecstasy from other sensual stimulators and social perceptions.

Probing beyond the young women's initial accounts of the culture as one in which sex did not feature also revealed a number of other sexual elements and experiences. The following are typical accounts of sexual experiences which respondents situated firmly within the context of the sexual safety they associated with the culture:

> It was great because I was at a rave and there was no sort of chance of having sex or anything and it was quite a secure sort of thing, more like I just sat in the corner and snogged for quite a long time and being cuddled and massaged and stuff and it was lovely ... I think it's [being on 'E' at a rave] just such a great big outburst of emotion than other emotions involved when you have sex, it would just have been far too much of a complex experience.
>
> (19-year-old student)

> We do fancy blokes at raves and enjoy flirting with them ... but it's like going back to when you were younger, you don't want to get them into bed, you're just friendly.
>
> (23-year-old computer analyst)

There were also descriptions of situations where young women had met young men in this context and thought them 'the best thing since sliced bread', exchanged phone numbers, saw them in another context and 'had nothing at all in common'. The sensuality/sexuality confusion expressed above also, in some cases, caused jealousy in relationships:

> My group of friends up here are all mixed and we all go out and we just have a good time and that's the end of it. I've known people last year that were actually seeing each other and had extreme problems going out together and doing E's because I mean you get all luvdup and you just see someone and you just want to hug them and be with them all night and you used to get boyfriend or girlfriend getting really jealous.

> (19-year-old student)

At least half the sample made reference to another component of the culture clearly relating to sexuality – that of sexual identity. Such references fell into two main categories: those which related generally to the blurring of sexual identity within the culture and the more specific references to an evident crossover between gay and heterosexual club culture which had resulted from the dance scene (see also Matthews, 1993). These features of at least certain sectors of the 'scene' clearly made an important contribution to its attraction for the young women concerned. These young women found gay culture both exciting and enjoyable on the grounds that, as before, the night's entertainment did not involve a predictable sexual narrative. Most of them had frequented gay clubs prior to becoming involved in the dance scene and singled out 'Flesh', the gay night at the time at Manchester's club the Hacienda, as a particularly enjoyable event in their clubbing calendar.

A number of accounts indicated the relaxation of heterosexual codes in the dance scene:

> It's always been affectionate, hugging and kissing girls you never met before like they're your lifelong friend, but recently you can see girls grinding together. A year ago, they would have been called lezzies or something but now nobody bats an eyelid.

> (22-year-old, unemployed)

> You see lots of lads hugging each other, a lot . . . sometimes they hug for so long you think 'when's the big snog coming?'

> (23-year-old computer consultant)

Some young lesbians and gay men also appear to feel more comfortable about seeking night-time recreation in sexually mixed settings. They also felt the scene had created a new social pace for young lesbians and gay men:

> I think a lot of women that do Es are into enjoying themselves in different ways and know how to have a good time and know that having a good time isn't shuffling about to Erasure at [a lesbian venue] and having a fight with a pool cue, you know. I think it does take out a lot of that crap and I think

there are a lot of dykes that have been looking for something that is a bit different.

(22-year-old DJ)

Younger guys are going straight on to the rave scene and leaving the high-energy scene down to the guys who are into the cruising scene . . . It's taken the seriousness out of it for a lot of boys I think. A lot of them feel safer and a lot less worried about being cruised by a man while they're out. Going out for a good time rather than just to cop off. It's totally changed the scene, split it in a lot of ways.

(22-year-old council administrator)

THE ROLE OF YOUNG MEN

The role played by young men in defining the sexual parameters and dynamics of the culture must, in the absence of other studies, be pieced together from the young women's accounts and other sources. Its importance should not be underestimated since the predominant image of young men's behaviour arising from the young women's accounts is one which differs from the more traditional one of young men in nightclubs intent upon pursuing sex. More interest in dancing, in physicality and interaction with young women without overt sexual intent, all featured widely in descriptions of male behaviour and a consequent preference on the part of the young women was for social environments in which this was the norm. This young man's private response to the sexual advances of a female new to the 'scene' who misread the sexual codes in a post-rave scenario, is typical of many: 'Doesn't she know we don't do that?'

If these features of male behaviour were an important defining feature of the culture for young women, the extent to which the pharmacological effects of specific drugs were the primary cause is less clear. Leaving aside the much-debated question of broader recent changes in perceptions of masculinity, two primary factors determining this male behaviour were foremost in the data. First, the effects associated with Ecstasy in general and on the male genitals in particular (shrinkage and inability to achieve erection). Second, the more general effect of often large dosages of psychedelic and stimulant drugs on male sexual interest. Distinguishing between these factors and the possible effects of the overall social and sexual codes prevalent within the culture on male behaviour is an impossible task, confounded by clear evidence of exceptions to this overall picture of male behaviour and sexuality in particular. While the young women took care to differentiate between 'beer monsters', who they saw to be intruders onto the 'scene', and the young men involved in the 'scene', the combination of possible factors did not diminish the male sexual imperative in all cases.

SEXUAL RISK

While the broader set of relationships between drugs and sexuality described above is illuminating, the question of drug-related sexual risk taking still remains. There was some indication that the 'scene' was not without sexual risk taking, but the precise role of drug use is unclear. Further probing during interviews yielded accounts of more traditional 'after club' casual sex scenarios. Interestingly, these were always recounted as general observations or as something only acquaintances involved themselves in. The fact that these were accurate descriptions was borne out not only by the exceptionally frank and relaxed atmosphere of the interviews but also by the of personal accounts of sexual risk taking which were offered.

Sexual risk taking under the influence

Two respondents gave accounts of an isolated case in which they had put themselves at risk while in a club context and under the influence of drugs. In both cases, the individuals concerned had taken three or more tablets of Ecstasy and regularly 'topped up' with amphetamine sulphate during the course of the night. The first involved a 20-year-old who later gave up the drugs and the 'scene' due to acute depression and anxiety. She described a situation in which she went to a private part of the club and had sexual intercourse with a door security man. The second described her experience thus:

> I got off with some bloke in a toilet at a rave not especially successfully, I was very ... I don't really know how I ended up in the toilet. I didn't really particularly know what was going on.
>
> (24-year-old librarian)

Both young women clearly felt they had been out of control at the time, had unprotected sexual intercourse and did not repeat the experience. Any interpretation suggesting that they might have conveniently explained their sexual risk taking as a result of heavy drug use has to be balanced by the fact that they were both consistently heavy users for a sustained period of time.

Sex and the 'comedown' period

Once again, the general ethos concerning the period after the club/party during which the drug effects are wearing off is that friends remain together in a range of relevant locations to 'chill out' – generally involving much smoking of cannabis. However, while the findings bear this out, they also suggest that this was the period during which sexual activity was most likely to take place, and under one of the following conditions: people 'chilling out' sometimes slip into sex out of boredom while waiting to be able to sleep;

couples go home and rest for a while, try and sleep and then, after smoking some draw, might try sex; and 'coming down' is seen by some as an ideal opportunity to 'smoke a load of draw and have lots of sex'.

This young woman's experience provides a possible explanation:

Of course the next day when you come down is a different matter, because you definitely feel horny. Partly because you go for a bit of comfort, it's the comfort you like and need on a Sunday when you're coming down.

(20-year-old administrator)

This young woman explained an unlooked-for sexual opportunity:

I took an 'E' that had no effect at . . . about 10–10.30 p.m. I suppose, went out and had a nice night anyway and just thought well that was a waste of money, and at 4.00 a.m. I came up . . . and I happened to be staying at my boyfriend's house so we'd gone to bed and it was absolutely wonderful, because with E you feel so much more, I mean anything, the clothes you wear feel wonderful when you wear them, when someone strokes you it feels wonderful because you are just so much more sensitive, so for a start, it means orgasms happen hundreds of times without you trying really, you don't have to do anything, you can talk dirty to me and that would be fairly exciting and it was quite amazing . . . . It was my perfect dream really because it was always that wonderful thing like, I'm going to be able to have millions of orgasms and he's not going to be able to have one, because that's so unusual because if you talk to a lot of women I think that's what they would like to inflict on a lot of men because so many men seem to think that the female orgasm was just as obtainable as the men so they don't bother to ask and find out.

(20-year-old student)

Perhaps more worrying was another young woman's account of her first time on Ecstasy with an older boyfriend experienced in drug taking. However, her account also suggests that such occurrences are indeed the exception rather than the rule:

I must admit I had sex with Andy after the first night at [a club venue]. At that point I didn't even know 'E' was supposed to make you feel horny. I felt quite loved up I must admit and I didn't regret it. Since then we've never had sex when we've been off our heads and I must admit it's got a lot better!

(15-year-old school student)

Drug use as a consciously chosen sexual enhancer

The young women also reported occasions when they had consciously chosen to experiment with Ecstasy with a sexual partner in a domestic context. These were exceptional cases and appeared to be confined, with one exception, to a single occasion of experimentation. This 22-year-old respondent had experimented with sex under the influence of what appeared to be high-quality Ecstasy on a number of occasions. Her account of the associated effects, on the whole, compares favourably with the others and was notable for the perceived advantage of having the opportunity to experiment with non-penetrative sex (perceived as a direct result of the effects of Ecstasy on male sexual organs) and delayed male and female orgasm. Other attempts were, however, described as 'a failure'. This would seem to be due largely to feelings of anxiety and paranoia which respondents felt had possibly been induced by the poor quality of the drug or more general over-indulgence in drug taking at the time.

IMPLICATIONS FOR HIV PREVENTION

These findings raise important implications for HIV prevention initiatives relating to gender, the relationship between drugs and sexuality and the role of popular culture in the harm reduction process.

Drugs and sexuality

The research gives both a much broader and more specific account of the relationship between drugs and sexuality than existing accounts: broader in that it maps the sexual codes and mores within which drug taking is conducted, more specific in the sense that it focuses on a specific culture of drug use. Both of these accounts contribute to an important basis for understanding sexual risk taking in a drug context. Although the precise role of the effects of Ecstasy and other drugs in determining the sexual codes within the culture is difficult to ascertain, the enhancement of sensual experience for women and diminishment of the imperative to seek sex among young men would appear to be key factors in determining what seems to be the lower level of risk taking within this environment compared to other cultures of recreational drug use.

Where sexual risk taking does occur, however, the perception of the general ethos of the 'dance drug' culture as being contrary to sexual partner-seeking can give rise to an element of surprise/non-preparation which could lead to non-protection. The 'comedown' period is the most likely time during which sexual risk taking is likely to occur but this period is also perceived by some as an opportunity to engage in 'planned' sexual activity of a safer nature. These factors, together with the continued popularity of the 'dance drug' phenomenon, its continual transformation and the consequent openness to change of the predominant relationships between sexuality and drug taking within it, suggest the need for continued attention. This is not least because a social setting within which young women's sexual and social options and choices appear to be less constrained by traditional gender norms than customary accounts suggest, provides an important basis for future development. More comparative studies of a similar nature which focus on different cultures of recreational drug use could also usefully build on these findings and provide an important basis for policy prioritisation.

Extending the repertoire of femininity

The resulting account of young women's involvement in 'dance drug' use and female sexuality in that context demonstrates that existing perspectives on both female drug use and young female sexuality are limited. While some attempt has been made to situate female drug use in its social context, the predominant view of the female user of illicit drugs as deviant or as a passive victim of a variety of social and psychological factors, has tended to militate against analyses open to the possibility that active female participation and contingent personal power and choice, within the confines of social constraints, are both possible and can be experienced by young women. Similarly, although some accounts of young female sexuality in the post-AIDS era have powerfully illustrated the gender dynamics of sexual negotiation, the predominant view of young female sexuality as lacking in pleasure and power remains largely intact (Holland et al., 1993).

By contrast, the research suggests that young women, on the whole, perceive their 'dance drug' taking as a pleasurable recreation and value a number of aspects of the total experience, its overall sensual, and often sexual, nature among them. The fact that these young women's wider sexual options and choices appear to be bound by constraints described elsewhere (Holland et al., 1993) underlines the importance of the 'dance drug' culture, both in terms of allowing the young women a social space within which their options and choices, sexual and otherwise, are increased and as a specific cultural setting within which important changes in gender relations are potentially lived out. Initiatives based on the assumptions of previous research – that women are powerless and unable to initiate their own pleasure, for instance – would fail to connect with the young women's self-perception and therefore be likely to fail entirely.

Young women and information needs

A number of suggestions regarding the content and form of information messages which could usefully target relevant young women were suggested by the research. While the young women were clearly actively involved in drug taking and often appeared to participate on grounds equal to young men, there were also important gender differences which suggest the need to ensure that health information reaches them. Drug information messages aside, a number of sexual health issues which occur in the context of drug use need to be covered. Concerns about the relationship between drug use and the menstrual cycle, contraception and pregnancy need to be addressed, as well as safer-sex messages relating to the drug-using context which, although they should target both sexes, would benefit from a gender-specific advice component.

The mode of delivering these messages is, however, all-important. The project's evaluation of Lifeline information materials (Henderson, 1993a) suggested that targeting young women with health messages is a more complex process than sometimes perceived. However sophisticated the approach, the use of a range of styles and formats would appear to be necessary since it is possible that no particular type of humour or visual form will appeal exclusively in gender terms. Humour and visual form seem to be highly efficient elements of communicating health messages in this context, matched only by the importance of 'source credibility' (Linnell, 1993) or the ability to demonstrate a familiarity with the norms and codes of the culture.

'Community' as a site for research and intervention

The project resembled other community-based HIV-related initiatives in its combination of ethnographic (and other) research methods with more practical distribution elements and its ongoing involvement of the 'researched' in the research and intervention process (see Chapter 12). However, it differed in a number of important respects. The target population were relatively easy to reach, were open about their drug use, and their lifestyles differed markedly from those of regular injectors. The definition of community which implicitly informed the project also differed markedly from the more explicit definitions central to community-based initiatives. 'Communities' for such intervention have been largely defined in terms of geographical location, social position, personal identity or specific shared behaviour. By contrast, the social structures working to define the target population as a 'community' in this case were largely commercial in nature – predominantly sectors (mainstream or 'alternative') of the media and leisure industries. This raises interesting and important questions for community-based prevention approaches, since the strong anti-consumerist ethic espoused by the earlier community development perspectives upon which they draw has been inherited to some degree. While they may not, like some earlier community development models, posit the restoration of 'real' human experience as an antidote to the ravages of consumer capitalism, such approaches are nonetheless presented as diametrically opposed and preferable to mass media approaches to prevention.

Popular culture as a site for intervention

The 'dance drug' phenomenon lends itself very well to the use of its cultural components for the circulation of harm reduction messages since there are so many associated outlets – bars, nightclubs and other venues, cafes, clothes and record shops, specialist magazines – and so many associated consumer products. Two drug agencies in the north-west of England have been notable for their interventions in the 'dance drug' phenomenon – the Lifeline Project in Manchester and the Mersey Drug Training and Information Centre (now HIT) in Liverpool. Both have been effective in communicating with their target audience and both have built their information campaigns on the vital foundation of a familiarity both with the norms and codes of the culture in question (from behaviour appropriate to different settings, to clothes styles, 'in' phrases and idioms, and changes in the type of drugs available) and with pertinent developments in the drug literature. The 'source credibility' of this form of communication (Linnell, 1993) has been achieved in different ways: Lifeline's use of humour and the development of a character – 'Peanut Pete' – in cartoon format and HIT's visual mimicry of the 'rave' flyer in the leaflet 'Chill Out' (McDermott et al., 1993). In their 'DAISY' campaign of summer 1993, however, HIT developed this model of communication by attempting to become part and parcel of the consumer culture associated with the dance drug phenomenon in Liverpool city centre. A range of consumer products already existing in the culture – including flyers, clothing swing labels, matches and cassettes cases – were used in the campaign. Distributed over a nine-week period in bars, cafes, clothes and record shops and publicised in national magazines associated with the culture, the campaign also utilised modern advertising techniques which actively engage their target audience in deciphering (initially mysterious) messages. It was highly effective in communicating with a 'community' defined in terms of a consumer lifestyle (Henderson, 1994b).

CONCLUSION

In the context of discussing the findings of research on the 'dance drug' phenomenon, this chapter has raised a number of considerations for future community-based prevention initiatives. First is the importance of flexibility in the understandings of gender brought to studies of health behaviours and to prevention initiatives. The assumption that, for instance, young women lack agency in the context of drug use and/or sexual encounters is clearly inadequate. Second, the relationship between drug use and sexuality, particularly sexual risk, is by no means a simple one and requires closer examination of the relationship between the social, pharmacological and situational factors involved and a brief broader than the current focus upon injecting drug use and sexual encounters. Finally, the repertoire of effective community-based initiatives has been extended by the development of a model which combines ethnographic techniques as a tool for becoming conversant with a specific culture, with the transmission of harm reduction messages via its key cultural components. In the case of the 'dance drug' culture, its many associated consumer products and outlets provide a ready-made vehicle for prevention.

REFERENCES

Balding, J. (1994) *Young People and Illegal Drugs, 1989–1995: Facts and Predictions*, University of Exeter: Schools Health Education Unit.

Blenheim Project (1989) *Changing Gear: A Book for Women Who Use Drugs Illegally*, London: Blenheim Project.

Broom, D. and Stevens, A. (1991) 'Doubly deviant', *International Journal on Drug Policy*, 2 (4): 25–27.

Buffum, J. and Moser, C. (1986) 'MDMA and sexual function', *Journal of Psychoactive Drugs*,18 (4):353–359.

Cuskey, W. (1982) 'Female addiction: a review of the literature', *Journal of Addictions and Health*, 3 (1): 3–33.

Dorn, N., Henderson, S., and South, N. (1992) *AIDS: Women, Drugs and Social Care*, London: Falmer Press.

Ettorre, E. (1992) *Women and Substance Use*, Basingstoke: Macmillan Press.

Ford, N. (1990) *Psychoactive Drug Use, Sexual Activity and AIDS Awareness of Young People in Somerset*, University of Exeter: Institute of Population Studies.

Henderson, S. (1990) *Women, HIV, Drugs: Practical Issues*, London: ISDD.

—— (1993a) *Young Women, Sexuality and Recreational Drug Use*, Final report, Manchester: Lifeline Project.

—— (1993b) 'Time for a makeover', *Druglink*, September/October: 14–16.

—— (1993c) 'Keep your bra and burn your brain', *Druglink*, November/December: 10–12.

—— (1993d) 'Fun, fashion and frisson', *International Journal on Drug Policy*, 4 (3): 122–129.

—— (1994a) 'Women and drugs in the context of AIDS', in L. Doyal, T. Wilton and J. Naidoo (eds) *AIDS: Setting a Feminist Agenda*, London: Falmer Press.

—— (1994b) *DAISY: An Evaluation of a Drug Information Campaign*, Liverpool: Mersey Drug Training and Information Centre.

Holland, J., Ramazanoglu, C., Scott, S., Sharpe, S., and Thomson, R. (1992) 'Pressure, resistance, empowerment: young women and the negotiation of safer sex', in P. Aggleton, P. Davies and G. Hart (eds) *AIDS: Rights, Risk and Reason*, Falmer Press: London.

Holland, J., Ramazanoglu, C., and Sharpe, S. (1993) *Wimp or Gladiator: Contradictions in Acquiring Masculine Sexuality*, WRAP/MRAP Paper 9, London: Tufnell Press.

ISDD (1994) *National Audit of Drug Misuse in Britain*, London: ISDD.

Lewis, L. (1991) 'Drug use and sex at dance parties in Sydney: a qualitative analysis', unpublished paper, National Centre in HIV Social Research Unit, University of New South Wales.

Linnell, M. (1993) *An Evaluation of Smack in the Eye*, Manchester: Lifeline Project.

McDermott, P., Matthews, A., O'Hare, P., and Bennett, A. (1993) 'Ecstasy in the United Kingdom: recreational drug use and subcultural change', in N. Heather, A. Wodak, E. Nadelamnn and P. O'Hare (eds) *Psychoactive Drugs and Harm Reduction: From Faith to Science*, London: Whurr.

McKeganey, N. and Barnard, M. (1992) *AIDS, Drugs and Sexual Risks. Lives in the Balance*, Buckingham: Open University Press.

Matthews, J. (1993) 'Into the unknown', unpublished dissertation, Manchester Metropolitan University.

Measham, F., Newcombe, R., and Parker, H. (1993) 'The post-heroin generation', *Druglink*, May/June: 16–17.

Mixmag (1992) Editorial, 2 (16): 2

Nasmyth, P. (1985) 'Ecstasy (MDMA)', *The Face*, 66.

Oppenheimer, E. (1991) 'Alcohol and drug misuse among women – an overview', *British Journal of Psychiatry*, 158 (10): 36–44.

Parker, H., Measham, F., and Aldridge, J. (1995) *Drug Futures*, London: ISDD

Perry, L. (1979) *Women and Drug Use: An Unfeminine Dependency*, London: ISDD.

Redhead, S. (ed.) (1993) *Rave Off: Politics and Deviance in Contemporary Youth Culture*, Aldershot: Avebury.

Rhodes, T. and Stimson, G. (1994) 'What is the relationship between drug taking and sexual risk? social relations and social research', *Sociology of Health and Illness*, 16(2): 209–229.

Rosenbaum, M. (1981) *Women on Heroin*, New Brunswick, NJ: Rutgers University Press.

Roth, P. (ed.) (1991) *Alcohol and Drugs Are Women's Issues*, Metuchen, NJ and London: Women's Action Alliance and the Scarecrow Press.

Sargent, M. (1991) 'Changing the paradigm: drugs in society', *National Women and Drugs Conference Proceedings*, Melbourne, 18–48.

—— (1992) *Women, Drugs and Policy in Sydney, London and Amsterdam*, Aldershot: Avebury.

Smash Hits (1992) 'Get sorted', 14–27 October:15–19.

the *Sun* (1988) 'The Evil of Ecstasy', 1 October.

Taylor, A. (1993) *Women Drug Users*, Oxford: Clarendon Press.

Thom, B. (1991) 'Women and substance misuse – reflections on becoming a "high-risk" group', paper to Women and Drugs Conference, Institute of Psychiatry, London.

Waterson, J. and Ettorre, E. (1989) 'Providing services for women with difficulties with alcohol or other drugs: the current UK situation as seen by women practitioners, researchers and policy makers in the field', *Drug and Alcohol Dependence*, 24: 119–125.

Wight, D. (1993) 'Constraints or cognition: factors affecting young men's practice of safer heterosexual sex', in P. Aggleton, P. Davies, and G. Hart (eds) *AIDS:Facing the Second Decade*, London: Falmer Press.

Wodak, A. (1990) 'Alcohol and women's health: a cause for concern?', *Health Right*, 9 (3): 17–22.

Chapter 6

Gay community oriented approaches to safer sex

Graham Hart

It is now well established from studies of gay and bisexual men in the USA, Europe and Australia that in the mid to late 1980s there was a major move towards the adoption of 'safer sex' in this population (Hart, 1989). However, while these trends may have applied on a population basis, unsafe sex was and remains a significant problem. Indeed, there has been an increase in the incidence of rectal gonorrhoea (taken as a proxy marker of unsafe sexual behaviour) in gay men in London (Singaratnam *et al.*, 1991), a rising incidence of HIV-1 infections in gay men (Evans *et al.*, 1993) and a continuing high prevalence of infection in gay and bisexual men in England (Hart *et al.*, 1993).

Evidence from the Day report (Communicable Disease Report [CDR], 1993) suggests that the epidemics of HIV infection and AIDS are set to continue in the UK among men who have sex with men (MSM), rising to an estimated annual incidence of 1,505 AIDS cases by 1997 in men for whom transmission occurred through homosexual intercourse. This figure is based on current estimates of the number of men who are currently infected with HIV who will go on to develop AIDS-defined disease. The back projections for HIV incidence are approximately five hundred per annum between 1986 and 1991. This means that the situation will get worse in terms of AIDS in gay men – many of whom became infected in the early to mid-1980s – and MSM will remain at high risk of contracting and transmitting HIV.

It is in this context that the prevention of HIV infection in gay men – which has been vital since the outset of the epidemic – takes on ever greater significance in the UK, and in the developed world generally. To date, health education for this group, whether from non-statutory or statutory agencies, has been predominantly individually focused, the emphasis being on inform-ation-giving approaches, with occasional acknowledgement of the value of self-empowerment (Aggleton, 1989). While these approaches have un-doubtedly played a major role in increasing levels of knowledge about HIV, its transmission and the means by which to protect oneself, there is little evidence to suggest a direct relationship between the provision of such information and either individual or population-based behaviour change

(AIDS Strategic Monitor: 1991; AIDS Strategic Monitor: Gay Bars, 1991). Indeed, it may be that the primary reasons for the move towards safer sex in gay men lie elsewhere, with information provision a necessary but not sufficient prerequisite for behaviour change.

Absent from the practice and research literatures until relatively recently have been accounts of community oriented models of HIV prevention. That is, prevention which depends upon the organised and deliberate harnessing of social networks to establish group norms and collective action to promote safer sex. This is surprising in that the epidemic of HIV/AIDS in gay men is the longest established – the disease was first seen in this group – and disproportionately affects MSM in the developed world. This chapter will explore the reasons for the relative absence of community oriented approaches from the social, epidemiological and behavioural literature on gay men, describe some community-based interventions, and end by considering the prospects for the development of future community oriented approaches to HIV prevention in this group. The chapter will begin with a discussion of the limitations of individualistic practice and research paradigms in order to establish why community oriented approaches are currently viewed so optimistically in terms of their potential to deliver the health dividend of protection against HIV infection.

INDIVIDUAL AND SOCIAL EXPLANATIONS

To date, many of the studies of gay male sexual behaviour take the individual as the focus of research (Hart and Boulton, 1995). Even though research data are reported on a group basis, with situational factors (broadly defined) varying within and between studies, the primary aim of most research has been to describe the particular characteristics of 'at risk' individuals. These can be demographic (age, geographic location, ethnicity), socio-economic (income, education, housing tenure), behavioural (reported sexual activity, use of alcohol/drugs), psychological (self-efficacy, depression, locus of control) and, on occasions, contextual (sex in bathhouses, by partner type, with condoms un/available). Analysis takes the form of the selection of unprotected anal intercourse or known HIV infection as the dependent variable(s), with cross-tabulations and multiple logistic regression models identifying which of the selected independent variables amongst those investigated correlate with or predict increased risk (e.g. young, poor, black, drug users with low self-esteem having sex with casual partners in public sex settings).

It is perhaps understandable that studies concerned with risk exposure are individually oriented because risk is concerned with actual or potential harm associated with specific activities or 'external' influences (which could be environmental or biological) but which have individual consequences. However, regardless of the nature of risk exposure we know that it is by no means randomly distributed throughout the population. In the case of HIV it was not necessarily gay men's individual characteristics which determined their increased risk, but rather their membership of a social group in which sexual mixing occurred at a level such that, once HIV became established, rapid spread was facilitated.

The major criticism of individually oriented approaches is that they have generally failed to recognise that it is social structural location and group membership which are of primary significance in determining sexual risk exposure and that it is the social conditions which facilitate the development of norms which make risky sexual practices possible, rather than the psycho-social make-up of individuals *per se*. Thus, while individuals become infected with HIV – and the personal consequences of this are overwhelming in their meaning and intensity (Richardson and Bolle, 1992) – the 'cause' of this is not exclusively to be found in a person's degree of self-efficacy or locus of health control, but in the social and epidemiological opportunities for exposure to HIV.

Studies in the UK have consistently questioned the applicability of psycho-social health behaviour paradigms such as the Health Belief Model and Health Locus of Control to gay male sexual risk activity (Fitzpatrick *et al.*, 1989; Hart *et al.*, 1992; Davies *et al.*, 1993). These models assume un-restricted volition in individuals to choose a 'rational' health behaviour in response to a particular health threat, and in so doing take no note of at least three broader influences on health behaviour and risk exposure. The first is the context of the sexual encounter itself – notably the partner(s) with whom sex takes place, and the immediate circumstance of that sexual episode. Second, there is the relationship of power evident in the sexual encounter, which can involve something approaching equality or any other interpersonal variant of power imbalance up to and including use of violent force including rape. Finally, there is the broader socio-structural context of the sexual exchange, and its direct effect on the form and content of sexual acts. Yet, with the exception of the first, these areas have rarely been investigated fully in relation to gay men, even though their value in studying other populations is evident (Hart and Boulton, 1995). A brief consideration of each of these areas will indicate their significance for understanding the social dimensions of risk exposure to HIV.

One of the most striking and consistent findings of behavioural research on gay men is that high-risk sex is more frequently reported with someone described as a 'regular' partner or lover (Hunt *et al.*, 1992; Hart *et al.*, 1993). In our own study of 677 homosexually active men (McLean *et al.*, 1994), we found that the main difference between regular and non-regular relationships was the degree of emotional involvement the respondents reported where unprotected intercourse in the context of a regular relationship was described as a way of expressing the love and commitment to a shared life that the men felt. The study demonstrates the significance of the affective context of the sexual encounter itself.

The second area of importance in sociological explanations of risk is to be found in the relationship of power evident in the sexual encounter. A good example of this is to be found in studies of male prostitution. Robinson and Davies (1991) contrasted the experiences of 'rent boys' – predominantly young working-class men, often not gay-identified who were involved in street prostitution and who offered sexual services as streetwalkers in central London – and 'call men' who worked from their own flat or an agency, were able to take clients home or could travel to clients' homes or hotel rooms, were often of middle-class backgrounds and self-identified as gay. Systematic differences between these two groups were observed in relation to risk behaviour, which in turn was related to differing access to material resources. Anal intercourse rarely took place between call men and their clients, and then it was usually with a condom, whereas penetration was much more common amongst rent boys and condom use intermittent. What this and similar studies indicate is the central role of material resources in constraining individual choice regarding risk behaviours (McKeganey et al., 1990; Davies et al.,1993).

Finally, there is the broader socio-structural context of the sexual exchange. Although in relation to gay men this dimension is ill-served with research, it should be noted that feminist researchers have identified gendered structures of inequality which have a direct bearing on sexual behaviour in heterosexual sex (Richardson, 1990; Wilton and Aggleton, 1991; Holland et al., 1991). In understanding sexual behaviour among gay, bisexual and other MSM there is increasing interest in critically exploring the effects of homophobic social policy such as in the restrictions on sex education in schools, the tardy and very limited state provision of health education for gay men, the clawing back of monies from HIV and AIDS services because there has been 'no heterosexual epidemic', and the legal restrictions placed on gay male sexuality. These suggest a reconsideration of homophobia not as a feature of individual personality, whether as pathology or attitude, but as a structured policy response (King, 1993). It may be challenging methodologically to suggest this as an area of research, connecting with lived experience and risk, but it is certainly not an area of study beyond empirical scrutiny.

In defence of the individualistic studies of gay men, however, it should be noted that in the last ten years they have succeeded in monitoring the progress of the epidemic. A reading of this literature indicates that the response by researchers to the HIV/AIDS epidemic in homosexual and bisexual men in the developed world has had three phases. In the first, researchers aimed to provide the basic epidemiological information which could help determine the degree of risk associated with particular activities, contexts and individuals (Goedert et al., 1984; McKusick et al., 1985). In the second phase, they demonstrated that gay men were able to make changes in their sexual behaviour and that this could result in substantial reduction in the absolute and relative rates of the transmission of HIV and other sexually transmitted diseases (Martin, 1987; Gellan and Ison, 1986). In the third, most recent and still developing, phase they have alerted us to the possibility of continuing infection as a result either of new risk behaviour by men just beginning their sexual careers or of systematic differences between men associated with socio-structural and cultural factors which militate against the adoption of safer sex (Stall *et al.*, 1990; Evans *et al.*, 1993).

However, the continuing individual focus of such research has also had negative consequences, notably in the unintended but evident pathologising of individual men as being prone to a weakening of the resolve to maintain safer sex and succumbing to the temptations of unprotected sex; in short, 'relapse'.

A CONSEQUENCE OF THE INDIVIDUAL FOCUS: 'RELAPSE'

A methodological feature of the large studies of gay male behaviour has been that, although usually reported as cross-sectional data, information often comes from participants in prospective cohort studies. The men are regularly approached to provide information on their most recent behaviour, which can then be compared to their earlier accounts. By undertaking such analyses it became clear to researchers that not all men had maintained safer sex. The term 'relapse' was introduced to describe the behaviour of that minority of men who had initially adopted safer sex behaviours but, at some point during follow-up, had had at least one episode of unprotected penetrative anal intercourse (Stall *et al.*, 1990). It appeared that a 'new' category of men had been uncovered – those who revert to their 'former' sexual ways in the later stages of the epidemic.

The methodological and conceptual bases of the concept 'relapse' have been criticised in detail elsewhere (Hart *et al.*, 1992; Davies, 1992), and a lively debate continues over the appropriateness of this term (Kippax *et al.*, 1993; Ekstrand *et al.*, 1993; Davies 1993). However, it is worth noting here in relation to risk behaviour that the term serves to encapsulate and express the individualised focus of much behavioural work in the AIDS field generally, and on gay men in particular. It is a term in common use in medicine, and particularly in the treatment of substance misuse, when periods of abstinence (where the person is 'drug free') may be followed by a return to the use of the drug of addiction. Indeed, in many dependency services, one-time alcoholics and drug dependent patients are subsequently described as being 'recovering alcoholics/drug addicts', with the expressed intention of indicating that they are always at risk of what in physical medicine would be called remission and here is referred to as 'relapse'. Outside medicine, the term is more clearly pejorative, and refers to back-sliding, or return to bad behaviour or states of being, and this is on the basis of individual and moral turpitude. Thus the use of 'relapse' is associated with pathology, and the state to which individuals return is couched in terms of disease. In relation to prevention, the result of this pathologising individualism is the recommendation to introduce interventions which target the 'morally weak' persons who cannot sustain safer sex (Hart *et al.*, 1992). Thus, in a recent campaign in San Francisco, gay men were challenged to identify 'excuses' for relapsing or engaging in any unsafe sex, and asked to call an AIDS counsellor at the end of a free phone-line who is undoubtedly there to challenge the individual transgressor to account for his behaviour (Watney, 1993).

The use of 'relapse', the assumptions that go along with it and the entire enterprise of engaging in individually focused studies are not 'wrong' in any practical sense, except that they unintentionally divert attention from other means of assessing and explaining sexual behaviours. They evidently do not engage in the much more difficult, yet important, enterprise of locating individuals in social networks and communities of interest, which can be studied to determine those features which encourage or militate against the adoption of safer sex. This involves introducing a perspective which does not make the individual an isolated unit acting without reference to his/her surroundings, other people or larger environment, but which accounts for risk activity precisely in terms of the person's immediate and broader social location and context. This paradigm does not deny human volition, or 'rationality', rather it asserts that human action (in this case, risk) is influenced by, and actively affects, involves, or has implications for, other people.

AN ALTERNATIVE APPROACH: COMMUNITY ORIENTED INTERVENTIONS

Although it was suggested earlier that few attempts have been made to establish community oriented models of HIV prevention among gay men, the history of the response of gay men to the epidemic is in fact one of community action (Patton, 1990; Watney, 1990). Organisations such as Gay Men's Health Crisis in New York, the Terrence Higgins Trust in the UK and Deutsche AIDS-Hilfe in Germany based their work upon struggles in the 1970s and early 1980s towards gay collective action and civil rights. These and similar organisations have their different histories and strategies, but all have achieved major gains despite recent criticism that they 'de-gayed' HIV by asserting that 'AIDS is everyone's problem' when it was and remains a primarily gay male epidemic in the developed world (King, 1993). Such organisations remain exemplars of successful collective action on the part of gay men and their allies, as they placed AIDS on the political and health agendas to the extent that today the epidemic remains a key health priority in developed countries. It is difficult to abstract lessons for other groups from the experience of gay men as there were quite distinctive features of both gay political action and perceptions of the disease which facilitated the development of a non-statutory response to AIDS. A predominantly middle-class and articulate pressure group, with access to politicians, liberal media and senior medics, was able to assert the need for targeted resources in the context of what was perceived as a particularly threatening phenomenon – a 'new' infectious disease in developed countries at the end of a century in which chronic non-infectious diseases are and remain the major cause of morbidity and mortality.

Although the development of gay-initiated non-statutory organisations both to provide and press for services for people threatened by or living with HIV disease is an example of gay community action, direct community oriented HIV prevention for gay men is not as widespread as is commonly assumed. Compared to other groups, such as drug users and sex workers, gay men may have achieved substantial gains through political organisation and lobbying, yet prevention of HIV infection has remained highly individualised, predicated upon personal behaviour change. This may be associated with the history of response to the epidemic as described above. First, the individualised orientation of much research on and health education for gay men by its nature militated against the adoption of community-based prevention. Second, the initially rapid collective response of key members of the gay community early in the epidemic was to put their energies into information campaigns for gay men and consciousness-raising regarding the threat of HIV/AIDS; subsequently they redirected their effort to all those at risk of HIV infection. Once gay men had been leafleted about HIV transmission and its avoidance and, later, presented with eroticised versions of safer sex, there was a health education hiatus in terms of future directions.

Recently this has changed, with substantial interest and active engagement in new approaches to the continuing problem of the exposure of gay men to HIV infection. This has come from community-based groups, gay men and their allies in health promotion and researchers with an interest in developing and evaluating different approaches to HIV prevention. In the following sections, work that has been undertaken in the USA and the UK will be described, although this is not intended to be an exhaustive review of all the community oriented prevention that is currently under way for gay and non-gay identified MSM.

Community oriented initiatives in the USA

In the United States, there have been the most systematic attempts both to initiate and to research community oriented approaches to HIV prevention among gay men. Two interventions in particular have generated a great deal of interest and are worth reporting in some detail. The first is the Men's Network, a community-level approach for young (18–28) gay men, in California. It is taking place in three medium-sized cities sequentially;

outcome data for one city were made available at the eighth International Conference on AIDS in Amsterdam (Kegeles *et al.*, 1992).

The 'network' of the title is made up of young gay men recruited from each of the cities, and the entire enterprise is peer-run and the programme peer-designed. Support is provided through the research budget for advertising materials and for the events that the men organise. The network is intended to be a dynamic body, with a turnover of members as people leave and new men are recruited. The programme itself consisted of peer outreach, which included formal presentations in bars and at community events – such as beach parties and discos – and by members of the network making informal contacts in popular cruising areas. Safer sex workshops were also organised.

Baseline data were collected six months before and then again immediately prior to the intervention, followed by questionnaires distributed immediately post-intervention, then six months later and again one year later. Preliminary findings were able to compare men 'highly exposed' (that is, who had participated in two or more events, were themselves network members or had attended workshops) and those 'not highly exposed'. The researchers found that there was a population-based increase in norms supporting safer sex, an increase in reported discussion with friends and more communication with sexual partners about safer sex; all of these were higher in the most exposed group. Reported enjoyment of unprotected sex fell in the highly exposed as compared to the less exposed group.

When first described, this research was at an early stage of development, but findings were promising. A major aim of the project was that it became self-perpetuating, through the constant turnover of members of the network and through the range of contacts made by the men *en masse* and individually. At the ninth International Conference on AIDS in Berlin, Tom Coates, one of the researchers involved in the project, favourably contrasted the effectiveness of peer-led initiatives, such as the three-city study, to one-off counselling in relation to safer sex, which has not been demonstrated to achieve long-term behaviour change or maintenance of safer sex (Higgins *et al.*, 1991).

The second intervention, and one of the most impressive for gay men, was first decribed by Kelly *et al.* (1991), also in relation to three cities, but by the time of the Amsterdam conference the programme had been extended to eight small cities in four states (Kelly *et al.*, 1992), and by the Berlin conference to sixteen cities (Kelly *et al.*, 1993). Cities were selected according to three criteria: they had a population of less than 250,000, were located at least sixty miles from any other city of the same or larger size, and each had a relatively discrete and identifiable gay male population, with between one and three well-used gay bars. Eight of the cities were randomly designated as intervention centres, and eight as comparators. In the comparison (control) cities high-quality AIDS education materials were introduced to and maintained in all of the gay bars throughout the period of the research, with materials changed every three months to maintain novelty. In the intervention cities a social norm/peer influence intervention was introduced. The conceptual model used was that of 'diffusion of innovation' (Rogers, 1983). This suggests that social norms – in this case in favour of safer sex – can be successfully introduced and diffused through a community when modelled, endorsed and communicated by popular opinion leaders or trend-setters.

Baseline sexual behaviour measures were taken of 4,500 men attending the bars in each of the sixteen cities. In the intervention cities bartenders were asked to identify gay men who were regular attenders at the bars and who were, in the opinion of the bartenders, well known, liked and respected by other men. These 'popular' men were approached by the researchers and recruited to a two-month training course on the transmission characteristics of HIV, safer sex behaviours, and conversational means of introducing topics such as sexual risk reduction. They then were asked to engage in conversations with at least fourteen different men attending bars, and others at private parties and elsewhere, over a five-week period, saying that they fully endorsed and had personally committed themselves to the practice and philosophy of safer sex. For example, in the intervention bars there would be posters on the walls representing traffic lights, and the 'popular opinion leaders' would wear similar badges; if asked about the badge, the opinion leader would use this as an opportunity to employ the analogy of the traffic lights to explain safer (green) and unsafe (red) sexual behaviours, making it clear that they had adopted safer behaviours. Although no city was denied educational materials, including posters, leaflets and videos, only the comparison cities were not exposed to the newly informed and enthusiastic peer educators – designated 'gay heroes'.

After three, six and nine months of study, repeat surveys were undertaken of men attending the bars in all cities. In the cities receiving the experimental intervention there were systematic reductions in population-based risk behaviour, with decreases from baseline measures of 20–25 per cent in the proportion of men reporting high-risk sex, and corresponding reductions in the reported frequency of such behaviour (Kelly et al., 1992). These data excluded the opinion leaders from analysis (around 10 per cent of the study populations) to determine the full effect on the target population. The researchers have also shown that this effect has been maintained over time, while further analysis demonstrated a dose-response, notably that men who attended the bars more often or participated in more conversations had greater decreases in risk behaviour than those less exposed to the conversations (Kelly et al., 1993). In the comparison (non-intervention cities) no significant risk reduction was found.

Both of the interventions described here – the 'Men's Network' and 'Gay Heroes' programmes – have their limitations, acknowledged by the researchers. The first is that the pre- and post-intervention surveys measure population-based rather than individual behavioural change. Thus, the projects do not demonstrate that specific individuals, followed over time, make the recommended changes; any measurable response is at the community level. Given that this is the aim of the interventions, this must be seen as an acceptable outcome, although the research design does not preclude the incorporation of individual exposure measures.

As demonstration projects using an essentially experimental design there are other considerations which relate to their wider applicability. For example, the criteria applied to the selection of both intervention and comparison cities in the 'Gay Heroes' study could not be applied in any other country outside North America as geographical propinquity and population size cannot be 'controlled' in the same way. In the UK, for example, relatively few cities – and certainly not sixteen – could be identified as candidates for either intervention or control status. Many gay men participating in a commercial gay scene who live in small towns and cities are willing to travel to larger urban centres offering a great deal more choice than one to three bars. These gay men are not so geographically isolated as those described in Kelly *et al.* 1992, and therefore are exposed to many influences in terms of their own and their peers' behaviour. Any such similar intervention attempted in the UK – if seeking to incorporate specified and measurable outcomes – would need to take this major factor into account.

Because at the time of reporting these were relatively recent interventions, the studies have yet to demonstrate effectiveness other than on measures of self-reported sexual behaviour. For example, the incidence of sexually transmitted diseases associated with unsafe sex other than HIV infection is a key indicator of sustained safer sex over time. If these projects were able to demonstrate a reduction in sexually transmitted diseases such as gonorrhoea, syphilis and acute hepatitis B infection in the intervention cities, this would be an additional and persuasive indication of success. Of course, the final and most significant outcome measure would be a reduced incidence of new HIV infections although, in areas with a relatively low prevalence and incidence of infection, it would be difficult if there is no increase in cases to attribute this exclusively to behavioural modification. The epidemiological and biological parameters of disease transmission are not so well-understood as to be entirely controllable in these experimental research designs.

There are other considerations. For example, the projects assume a large degree of cultural homogeneity between the cities studied in terms of their respective gay populations. Even if this obtains in US cities, will the same apply in other developed and developing countries? As demonstration projects, with substantial costs, what of subsequent financial and administrative support for those men who as members of networks or as peer leaders wish to continue the projects once research interest has abated? Will they be able to maintain the energy and enthusiasm so often reported in these studies? Can community norms, network effects and changes in identity – outcomes which have been claimed, either explicitly or implicitly – survive the possibly short-term effects of highly focused and discrete experimental interventions?

In the UK, most unsafe sex occurs in regular relationships rather than in casual encounters (Hart *et al.*, 1993; Davies *et al.*, 1993). Are these interventions equipped to deal with the often complex dynamics of personal relationships which may militate against the adoption of safer sex (Hickson *et al.*, 1992; Hart, 1993)? These and other questions arise, although it must be said that the originality, organisation and execution of these interventions are testimony to the commitment of all those involved, as members of social networks, opinion leaders and researchers.

Community oriented initiatives in the UK

Although a number of community oriented interventions have been tried in the UK, none has been subject to the same level of scrutiny as has occurred in the USA. Indeed, for the most part projects have been service driven, with little or no research attached to them. Studies that have taken place have been concerned mainly to describe the processes of setting up and running interventions with some reference to the numbers of men contacted and their satisfaction with the services, as opposed to establishing behavioural or epidemiological outcomes as in the US projects.

This is understandable. It is often very difficult to secure the most basic funding, for example to run workshops or provide training for identified peer leaders, and this becomes even more challenging when there are full- or part-time staff costs. As the funders of interventions rarely include a research element as part of a budget for services, those who are committed to the project then have to apply for research monies from other organisations, often in the absence of substantial research experience or expertise. So, whilst a great deal of enthusiasm for the intervention is evident, research is at best an afterthought and at worst simply not present as part of the intervention.

In other circumstances research has been included as part of the setting up of a project. For example, the non-statutory organisation Gay Men Fighting AIDS (GMFA) has secured funding from North West Thames Regional Health Authority to undertake a peer-led initiative among gay men called Stop-AIDS London, but has also been able to fund research on the project, undertaken by the Health Education Research Unit of the Institute of Education, University of London. These monies were allocated by North East Thames Regional Health Authority, which clearly considers that the project could have major London-wide implications.

To date, the most systematic account of community work intervention in the UK is to be found in Prout and Deverell (1995), although this focuses on one set of linked interventions – the men who have sex with men action in the community (MESMAC) projects – and was not intended to be a comprehensive survey of all community oriented approaches for gay men in the UK. Broadly speaking, the MESMAC projects fell into one of three major categories. These were groups organised for social and health activities (e.g.

Tyneside Gay Men's Youth Group), for outreach (e.g. Leicester Black MESMACs work in saunas) and to set up peer-led programmes (e.g. London MESMACs Peer Training Initiative). There were also one-off and specific projects such as Latex Productions, a lesbian and gay theatre group in Leeds, although initially this served a similar function to the social groups in that its effects were measured primarily in terms of group members rather than on audiences. Some of the groups (e.g. Latex Productions) are extant; others were wound up within a year of forming.

The MESMAC projects varied quite considerably in the extent to which HIV prevention was their primary goal. For example, the Tyneside Young Men's Group and Leeds' 'Fit Together' were concerned to address a broader range of issues in relation to sexuality, health and social support than HIV alone. This was done in different ways in the two locales: the Tyneside group provided primary support for young men's chosen sexuality, whilst the Leeds group functioned more as a coalition of individuals and organisations in a network with broadly shared health aims. Each organised HIV-related events or incorporated HIV-specific issues within their remit, but prevention was never the exclusive concern of group members.

The outreach organised in Leicester for Black MSM and the London Peer Training Initiative were more concerned to incorporate directly HIV-related prevention in their work, although again this took place in a framework that emphasised related issues of sexuality and sexual health. In Leicester the focus of work was saunas which were not gay identified but which were places where Asian, Afro-Caribbean and white men came to have sex with other men. Few of these men were involved in or wished to be a part of the commercial gay scene, and the MESMAC workers therefore worked with men on a one-to-one basis to provide information on sexual health issues, distribute condoms and discuss issues of sex and sexuality with men who did not normally have access to this kind of resource. In London the Peer Training Initiative had safer sex as its stated goal, through peer-led outreach in the community. Although training meetings were organised on HIV, safer sex and its negotiation, and on drug use issues, which reportedly benefited the ten members of the group who regularly came to meetings, the planned peer outreach work did not occur.

It is clear from this brief account of some examples of MESMAC projects that there has been substantial variation in the extent to which community development approaches to HIV prevention are demonstrably effective in stopping the further spread of HIV and other sexually transmitted diseases. The significant word here is 'demonstrably'. Even in those instances where HIV prevention was a primary goal, interventions were not developed in such a way that behavioural and epidemiological outcomes were incorporated as key measures in the evaluation of these services. In the MESMAC projects that were based on group work the research was primarily descriptive, with accounts of the process of recruiting and organising groups, and their effects on members. In the case of outreach projects, for example, in saunas and public toilets where sex between men takes place ('cottages'), the perceived difficulties of measuring effectiveness and the lack of resources for studying behavioural and other outcomes meant that the research was mostly concerned with evaluating the practicalities of service delivery, rather than its effects. MESMAC and its associated research was primarily an exercise in establishing that community development can be an organising principle and an achievable practice, rather than an attempt to demonstrate that one form of community development would succeed in HIV prevention, whereas another would not.

Some of the MESMAC projects have continued in a similar form, several have been abandoned, and others have developed into free-standing agencies or groups with their own agenda for future work. Other projects are starting up in many parts of the UK, but to date there have been no published accounts of collaborative ventures between service providers and researchers to develop demonstration projects along the lines of the US interventions described earlier: that is, where HIV prevention is perceived as a primary, if not exclusive, goal with the realisation of specific outcomes identified as evidence of effectiveness in achieving this goal. With HIV transmission showing little sign of abating among homosexually active men in the UK, there is ever greater urgency for such interventions to be established.

DISCUSSION

In this chapter I have described research and interventions in which the focus of both research and intervention is not, in the first instance, the individual gay man and his personal attributes which are then used to 'explain' whether safer sex is adopted. The concern here is not with health beliefs, locus of control, self-efficacy or 'relapse' – the armoury of concepts introduced which over-determine the individual as solely responsible for all risk taking in sexual contexts. The research reported here has recognised that factors other than the constituents of personal psychological make-up are important in our understanding of exposure to HIV infection.

It is possible to undertake interventions and research which recruit individual members of a particular group, and explore the contextual, power and socio-economic factors associated with particular behaviours. However, a different approach demands that one start not with individuals, but with the contexts in which they act. This is effected by directing research attention to the social relations connecting communities, groups and individuals and, in the case of sexual behaviour, social networks and dyads. The more difficult methodological lesson to be gained from a study of community oriented HIV prevention initiatives is one which demands that the researcher make, as a first step, a full investigation of the context in which risk activity occurs. On occasions this is made easier by spatial and temporal propinquity, although it is relatively rare in the developed world for gay men to live and work in the areas in which they socialise or have sex.

Questions must be asked about the nature of gay 'communities', their cohesion, support, accessibility and ease of entry. Kippax *et al.* (1992) in Australia found that men who had a strong gay identity were more likely to engage in safer sex than men on the periphery of or not engaging in an identifiable gay scene, who were not 'out' and whose primary public sexual identity was not gay. Again, these and other features of male same-sex activity may be crucial in understanding sexual risk taking, even though it may be empirically challenging to link such notions as 'homophobia' or 'gay community involvement' to individualised risk behaviour. Nevertheless, so rarely has it been attempted – beyond unsupported rhetoric which asserts rather than investigates such relationships – that taking up the challenge could prove extremely fruitful.

It is understandable that research on risk is individually oriented because the concept itself is so directly concerned with actual or potential harm associated with behaviour. Even within epidemiology, however, with its primarily medical (i.e. individual) focus it is understood that this is not necessarily as a result of individual human action, because environmental factors so often determine 'risk exposure'. Sociologists, unconstrained by an exclusively individual focus – indeed, spurred on by disciplinary imperatives to seek explanations beyond the level of the psyche, self or will – have both obligation and opportunity to explore the social dimensions of human relations and action, with the study of sexuality in particular offering many possibilities for the disclosure of the social dynamics of intimate and personal interactions. By understanding that sexual acts involving two or more people are examples of social action it becomes possible to determine the nature of any risk or hazard in terms of these primarily social relations. It is the expressed aim of community oriented health promotion for gay men to recognise that it is the links shared by and connecting participants, and the context in which activity occurs, that are significant. The social relations which further connect those involved to communities of interest within broader social structures should be the starting point rather than an after-thought for those who wish to study the social dynamics of risk.

REFERENCES

Aggleton, P. (1989) 'Evaluating health education about AIDS', in P. Aggleton, G. Hart and P. Davies (eds) *AIDS: Social Representations, Social Practices*, Brighton: Falmer Press.

AIDS Strategic Monitor (1991) *Report on the Survey Period November 1987–December 1988*, London: BMRB/HEA.

AIDS Strategic Monitor: Gay Bars (1991) *Report on a Quantitative Survey in Gay Bars, January–February 1990*, London: BMRB/HEA.

Communicable Disease Report (CDR) (1993) *The Incidence and Prevalence of AIDS:*

HIV Disease in England and Wales for 1992–1997: Projections Using Data to the End of June 1992, Report of a working group (Chairman: Professor N.E. Day), 3 (Supp. 1): S1–S17.

Davies, P. (1992) 'On relapse: recividism or rational response?', in P. Aggleton, P. Davies and G. Hart (eds) *AIDS: Rights, Risk and Reason*, Brighton: Falmer Press.

Davies, P. M. (1993) 'Safer sex maintenance among gay men: are we moving in the right direction?', *AIDS*, 7: 279–280.

Davies, P.M., Hickson, F.C.I., Weatherburn, P. and Hunt, A.J. (1993) *Sex, Gay Men and AIDS*, Brighton: Falmer Press.

Ekstrand, M., Stall, R., Kegeles, S., Hays, R., De May, M. and Coates, T. (1993) 'Safer sex among gay men: what is the ultimate goal?', *AIDS*, 7: 281–282.

Evans, B.G., Catchpole, M.A., Heptonstall, J., Mortimer, J.Y., McGarrigle, C.A., Nicoll, A.G. *et al.* (1993) 'Sexually transmitted diseases and HIV-1 infection among homosexual men in England and Wales', *British Medical Journal*, 306: 426–428.

Fitzpatrick, R., Boulton, M. and Hart, G. (1989) 'Gay men's sexual behaviour in response to AIDS', in P. Aggleton, G. Hart and P. Davies (eds) *AIDS: Social Representations, Social Practices*, Brighton: Falmer Press.

Gellan, M.C.A. and Ison, C.A. (1986) 'Declining incidence of gonorrhoea in London: a response to fear of AIDS?', *Lancet*, 2: 920.

Goedert, J.J., Biggar, R.J., Winn, D.M. *et al.* (1984) 'Determinants of retrovirus (HTLV-III) antibody and immunodeficiency conditions in homosexual men', *Lancet*, 2: 711–716.

Hart, G., (1989) 'AIDS, homosexual men and behavioural change', in C.J. Martin and D.V. McQueen (eds) *Readings for a New Public Health*, Edinburgh: Edinburgh University Press.

Hart, G. (1993) 'Safer sex: a paradigm revisited', in P. Aggleton, P. Davies, and G. Hart (eds) *AIDS: Facing the Second Decade*, Brighton: Falmer Press.

Hart, G. and Boulton, M. (1995) 'Sexual behaviour in gay men: towards a sociology of risk', in P. Aggleton, P. Davies and G. Hart (eds) *AIDS: Safety, Sexuality and Risk*, London: Taylor and Francis.

Hart, G., Boulton, M., Fitzpatrick, R., McLean, J. and Dawson, J. (1992) '"Relapse" to unsafe sexual behaviour amongst gay men: A critique of recent behavioural HIV/AIDS research', *Sociology of Health and Illness*, 14: 216–232.

Hart, G., Dawson, J., Fitzpatrick, R., Boulton, M., McLean, J., Brookes, M. and Parry, J.V. (1993) 'Risk behaviour, anti-HIV and anti-HBc prevalence in clinic and non-clinic samples of gay men in England, 1991–1992', *AIDS*, 7: 863–869.

Hickson, F., Davies, P. Hunt, A.J. *et al.* (1992) 'Maintenance of open gay relationships: some strategies for protection against HIV', *AIDS Care*, 4: 409–419.

Higgins, D.L., Galavotti, C., O'Reilly, K.R. *et al.* (1991) 'Evidence for the effects of HIV antibody counselling and testing on risk behaviors', *Journal of the American Medical Association*, 266: 2419–2429.

Holland, J., Ramazanoglu, C., Scott, S., Sharpe, S. and Thomson, R. (1991) 'Between embarrassment and trust: young women and the diversity of condom use', in P. Aggleton, G. Hart and P. Davies (eds) *AIDS: Responses, Interventions and Care*, Brighton: Falmer Press.

Hunt, A.J., Davies, P.M., McManus, T.J., Weatherburn, P., Hickson, F.C.I., Chrisofinis, G., Coxon, A.P.M. and Sutherland, S. (1992) 'HIV infection in a cohort of gay and bisexual men', *British Medical Journal*, 305: 561–562.

Kegeles, S., Hays, R., and Coates, T. (1992) 'A community-level risk reduction intervention for young gay and bisexual men'. Proceedings of VIII International Conference on AIDS/III STD World Congress, Amsterdam (PoD5749).

Kelly, J.A., St Lawrence, J.S., Diaz, Y.E., Stevenson, L.Y., Hauth, M.A. *et al.* (1991)

'HIV risk behavior reduction following intervention with key opinion leaders of population: an experimental analysis', *American Journal of Public Health*, 81: 168–171.

Kelly, J.A., Sikkema, K.J., Winett, R.A., Soloman, L.J., Roffman, R.E., Kalichman, S.C. and Stevenson, L.Y. (1992) 'Outcomes of a 16-city randomized field trial of a community-level HIV risk reduction intervention'. Proceedings of VIII International Conference on AIDS/III STD World Congress, Amsterdam (ToD 0543).

Kelly, J.A., Winett, R.A., Roffman, R.E., Soloman, L.J., Sikkema, K.J., Kalichman, S.C. *et al.* (1993) 'Social diffusion models can produce population-level HIV risk behaviour reduction: field trial results and mechanisms underlying change'. Proceedings of IXth International Conference on AIDS/IVth STD World Congress, Berlin (PO–C23–3167).

King, E. (1993) *Safety in Numbers*, London: Cassell.

Kippax, S., Crawford, J., Connell, B., Dowsett, G., Watson, L. *et al.* (1992) 'The importance of gay community in the prevention of HIV transmission: A study of Australian men who have sex with men', in P. Aggleton, P. Davies and G. Hart (eds) *AIDS: Rights, Risk and Reason*, Brighton: Falmer Press.

Kippax, S., Crawford, J., Davis, M., Rodden, P. and Dowsett, G. (1993) 'Sustaining safe sex: a longitudinal study of a sample of homosexual men', *AIDS*, 7: 257–263.

McKeganey, N.P., Barnard, M.A. and Bloor, M.J. (1990) 'A comparison of HIV-related risk behaviour and risk reduction between female street-working prostitutes and male rent boys in Glasgow', *Sociology of Health Illness*, 12: 274–292.

McKusick, L., Horstman, W. and Coates, T.J. (1985) 'AIDS and sexual behavior reported by gay men in San Francisco', *American Journal of Public Health*, 75: 4933–4936.

McLean, J., Boulton, M., Brookes, M., Lakhani, D., Fitzpatrick, R., Dawson, J., McKechnie, R. and Hart, G. (1994) 'Regular partners and risky behaviour: why do gay men have unprotected intercourse?', *AIDS Care*, 6: 331–341.

Martin, J.L. (1987) 'The impact of AIDS on gay male sexual behavior patterns in New York City', *American Journal of Public Health*, 77: 578–581.

Patton, C. (1990) 'What science knows: formations of AIDS knowledges', in P. Aggleton, P. Davies and G. Hart (eds) *AIDS: Individual, Cultural and Policy Dimensions*, Brighton: Falmer Press.

Prout, A. and Deverell, K. (1995) *MESMAC: Working with Diversity, Building Communities*, London: HEA/Longman.

Richardson, D. (1990) 'AIDS education and women: sexual and reproductive issues', in P. Aggleton, P. Davies and G. Hart (eds) *AIDS: Individual, Cultural and Policy Dimensions*, Brighton: Falmer Press.

Richardson, A. and Bolle, D. (1992) *Wise before Their Time*, London: HarperCollins.

Robinson, T. and Davies P. (1991) 'London's homosexual male prostitutes: power, peer groups and HIV', in P. Aggleton, G. Hart and P. Davies (eds) *AIDS: Responses, Interventions and Care*, Brighton: Falmer Press.

Rogers, E.M. (1983) *Diffusion of Innovations*, New York: Free Press.

Singaratnam, A.E., Boag, F., Barton, S.E., Hawkins, D.A. and Lawrence, D.A. (1991) 'Preventing the spread of HIV infection', *British Medical Journal*, 302: 469.

Stall, R., Ekstrand, M., Pollack, L., McKusick, L. and Coates, T.J. (1990) 'Relapse from safer sex: the next challenge for AIDS prevention efforts', *Journal of Acquired Immune Deficiency Syndromes*, 3: 1181–1187.

Watney, S. (1990) 'Safer sex as community practice', in P. Aggleton, P. Davies, and G. Hart (eds) *AIDS: Individual, Cultural and Policy Dimensions*, Brighton: Falmer Press.

Watney, S. (1993) 'Emergent sexual identities and HIV/AIDS', in P. Aggleton, P.

Davies, and G. Hart (eds) *AIDS: Facing the Second Decade*, Brighton: Falmer Press.

Wilton, T. and Aggleton, P. (1991) 'Condoms, coercion and control: heterosexuality and the limits to HIV/AIDS education', in P. Aggleton, G. Hart and P. Davies (eds) *AIDS: Responses, Interventions and Care*, Brighton: Falmer Press.

Chapter 7

Prostitution and peer education

Beyond HIV

Marina Barnard and Neil McKeganey

Concern over the presumed potential for prostitutes to act as a bridgehead for HIV infection to pass into the general population has led to the setting up of a number of HIV prevention services targeted specifically at prostitutes. Cynically one might argue that the concern expressed was less for the health and well-being of the prostitute than for the people she might pass infection on to. Nonetheless, the attention (and finance) directed at preventing potential HIV spread through prostitution has resulted in the provision of services specifically aimed at prostitutes enabling them to work more safely and to ensure their own health. Perhaps one of the few good things to come out of the AIDS epidemic has been the forced recognition of the health needs of groups of people (drug users, prostitutes, men who have sex with men) who are socially marginalised and who often remain hidden to services. The onerous task of preventing HIV spread has led to a number of welcome changes in the planning and delivery of services. In their efforts to attract a wider client base, services have had to become more innovative, less agency-based and more attuned to the varying needs of the people they are designed to serve.

However, times are changing. Heterosexually acquired HIV has not spread within the developed world in the dramatic way envisaged in many of the early projections. Moreover, in so far as prostitutes in Britain are concerned, HIV does not appear, at the moment, to be a significant issue. Studies in London and in Glasgow both identified low levels of HIV infection (Ward *et al.*, 1993; McKeganey *et al.*, 1992). The low prevalence of HIV infection among prostitutes in Britain, at least, has implications for the future of HIV prevention services. Certainly with public spending cuts it is at least likely that these services will come under increased financial pressure to cut back both on the range and quality of services on offer.

The point we shall make in this chapter is that whilst it may have taken an epidemic for the health needs of prostitutes to be recognised and attended to, these same needs do not disappear simply because HIV is not spreading in this population as was once thought. The public health concern with the risks posed by prostitutes to others needs now to be turned on its head to consider the risks of prostitution for those who engage in it. In this chapter we will consider ways in which prostitutes themselves would benefit from services and interventions. Most of the services instituted for prostitutes have been directed at the management and monitoring of their sexual health. However, there are other aspects of prostitution which are hazardous and have an impact on the overall health of individual women. These are considered, as are the interventions which might be devised to counter these hazards. In particular, we will argue the value of interventions which draw on the resources of the prostitutes themselves for their planning and implementation. We will also consider the practicalities of any such interventions. This chapter focuses on streetworking prostitutes as it is they who are arguably most in need of services. The data presented here are derived from a study we conducted among Glasgow streetworking prostitutes. This work has been described in detail elsewhere (McKeganey *et al.*, 1992, 1993; McKeganey and Barnard, 1992; Barnard 1992, 1993). For the purposes of this chapter, however, it is worth providing a brief summary of the study and the methods it employed.

A STUDY OF GLASGOW STREETWORKERS

It was in response to the uncertainty over the possible connections between prostitution and HIV spread that this work was funded. Women working as prostitutes were contacted in the Glasgow 'red light' district over a period of three years. During this time, we systematically covered the range of times that women were observed to be working over each day of the week. In each year of the study we were able to contact approximately 150 prostitutes. Women were contacted directly by the researchers who regularly visited all of the streets comprising the red light district. The research also incorporated service provision. Each woman contacted was routinely offered assorted condoms, sterile needles and syringes and an advice and information leaflet. The study was both epidemiological and sociological in scope. In terms of the former, we looked at the prevalence of streetworking prostitution in Glasgow (using capture/recapture techniques to estimate population size) and the prevalence of HIV infection in this population (analysing anonymised saliva samples provided by the women).

These data were complemented by the collection of detailed sociological information relating to the women's HIV-related risk behaviours. The data used to inform this chapter were largely derived from short informal street interviews which were carried out with as many of the women as possible. These were mostly concerned with aspects of their work and private lives which were potentially associated with HIV risk. In addition, we draw on information collected through semi-structured interviewing of women in their homes as well as observational data we individually recorded in field diaries throughout the fieldwork period.

SERVICES TO STREET PROSTITUTES: SAFER SEX IS NOT JUST ABOUT CONDOMS

Prostitutes have long been thought to be under-represented as users of sexual health clinic-based services. This may be because clinics have tended to operate during the day and may therefore be inconvenient to visit or because women are reluctant to face possible stigma through acknowledging their prostitution. The public health importance placed on contacting greater numbers of prostitutes has led to the development of services targeted specifically at working women. Services have been set up in areas known to be worked by prostitutes and, importantly, accessible at the times when prostitutes themselves would be working (McIver, 1992). Some services have been able to go beyond a narrow focus on genito-urinary medicine to attend more broadly to the health needs of prostitutes. So, for example, drug injecting prostitutes can have drug related infections such as abscesses treated. They can also have access to clean needles and syringes. Some services provide all prostitutes with inoculation against hepatitis B (Carr *et al.*, 1992). These services are particularly useful for those women involved in drug injecting as it they who are often least likely, or least able, to ensure adequate health care for themselves (Hepburn, 1992). Prostitutes appear to value these services for their ease of access and the non-judgemental approach of staff. Furthermore, many such services have also tried to go beyond a purely medical role by creating a relaxed social atmosphere where women can go to take a break, or find respite, from their work. Where services are not located at specific premises, outreach services have often been initiated to facilitate contact with prostitutes (Synn Stern, 1992; Matthews, 1990).

The services provided to prostitutes have generally focused on sexual health, particularly on HIV prevention. Providing women with assorted condoms and encouraging their use with clients is clearly of value. So too is it valuable for women to have access to genito-urinary clinical care in a setting where they do not feel judged for being involved in prostitution. There are, however, aspects of prostitution which have an impact on health and well-being but which present difficult challenges for services.

Safer sex has come to be seen as synonymous with condom use and, to a lesser extent, with non-penetrative sex. However, ensuring safer commercial sex is not simply a matter of providing condoms. As prostitutes know, it is also about the ability to negotiate condom use with clients or reach agreement about having other kinds of non-penetrative sex. Successful negotiation requires the skills and confidence to be assertive in relations with clients (Bloor *et al.*, 1993). The safer commercial sex encounter does not only concern the prevention of possible HIV transmission. Prostitutes are also concerned to prevent the possibility of violent attack by clients. Successful negotiation with the client over the provision of sexual services can also involve screening the client, making judgements about his likely cooperativeness and the possible danger he might represent.

The process of negotiation between prostitute and client appears to represent an important benchmark in the commercial sex encounter. It is at this stage that the prostitute has the opportunity to assert her terms and conditions of business, which includes such issues as condom use. This clearly suggests the value of intervention strategies targeted at increasing the success with which prostitutes are able to negotiate a safer commercial sex encounter. Before looking at possible interventions, it is worth considering the dynamics of negotiation between client and prostitute. Success in achieving and sustaining behavioural change must to an important extent be premised upon an understanding of existing behaviours (Shedlin, 1990).

THE PROCESS OF NEGOTIATION

The buying and selling of sex is not the same as other kinds of transaction if only because we, and the societies we are part of, have such deep-seated and often contradictory notions of sex and sexuality and its appropriate expression. Furthermore, it is difficult, if not impossible, to separate sex from issues of power and control. These can potentially become highly charged in the context of commercial sex.

Prostitutes, particularly those working on the street, have two main objectives. First they aim to secure payment from clients for services rendered. Second, they want that contact to be safe, which includes protection against HIV infection but also against rape, robbery or worse. To these ends, the women deliberately aim to adopt an assertive, businesslike stance in their contacts with clients. Prostitutes create the conditions for client compliance by setting the terms of the transaction as explicitly as possible. Immediately it is established that the man is looking to buy sex, the woman will state her prices for different sex acts. She will also state where she is prepared to provide sex as well as what sex she will agree to. Retaining some control over the commercial sex encounter often appeared to be closely linked with notions of personal safety. This seems clear from the following field extract:

> In response to an earlier query about whether it was she who was in control or the client, Anna musingly responded 'Y' know it probably is me who's in control.' I then asked if it would make her anxious if a client tried to take control; 'Aye, aye, aye. It would make me anxious 'cos if he wants to go to his place y'know, him saying "I know a place." No. He could have his pals there. See you've always got to have your mind alert to these. You've got to be, you've always got to be, as I say, one step ahead . . . as soon as you get in that motor you're vulnerable.'

The advantage clients often have over prostitutes is one of greater physical strength. This is compounded by the fact that in response to current legislation against prostitution, most commercial sex occurs in places which are dark and ill-frequented. Both factors inevitably exacerbate a prostitute's vulnerability in any potentially violent situation and further underline the importance of trying to gain client compliance, or to screen out those men who do not look likely to assent.

From the point when a man expresses interest in purchasing sexual services, prostitutes have to make a series of quick decisions: how much money he is likely to have; whether or not he is safe to go away with. While negotiation between prostitute and client is explicitly about the type of sex wanted, condom use, the price and the place, so also all this time the woman is looking for clues about the man and how advisable it is to go with him. Take for example the following instance where a woman had to weigh up a client's seemingly attractive offer:

Maddy told me about a punter she'd had asking for an 'all-nighter' in a hotel. 'I told him that'd be £40 at least, but he wouldnae. So, I thought, dodgy. I mean all you can do is get the money up-front and if you can't then you can't really take that chance.' She didn't want to go into the hotel room with him without the money because she felt uneasy about him and his motives. If she'd managed to get money from him she said she would have felt more sure of him.

Since it is in the nature of prostitution that most men will be complete strangers to the women and since women cannot prolong the negotiation period if they are to avoid attracting police attention, they have to rely heavily upon their intuitive skills. That these skills are not foolproof is demonstrated by the high levels of client violence reported by prostitute women (Barnard, 1993; Silbert, 1981).

Once agreement is reached, the woman will get into the car or go to an alleyway with the client, although her watchfulness does not cease with the acceptance of business. Once with a client, prostitutes interpret any deviation from their instructions as being potentially dangerous. Often this is sufficient reason for them to terminate their agreement to provide sexual services, if it is still possible for them to do so:

Tina was still really cross when we met up with her after having been messed around by punters. Two men had wanted to buy sex from her and her pal. Tina had been unsure. 'Y'know they looked dodgy, but she's goin' "c'mon, a punter's a punter", so I went.' She'd asked them to turn left. 'I was wantin' to go to that wee car park. I know there was two of us an' all but still . . .' Instead the car had carried right onto the motorway. At this point Tina told them to stop the car as she became alarmed by the driver's lack of compliance. She and her friend had then had to walk all the way back none the richer for their trouble.

Prostitutes have devised a number of strategies to defend against attack should clients turn nasty. Each of them has practical or legal constraints limiting their effectiveness. A common strategy was to ask other women to look out for them while they were with a client. This requires that the watching woman remain without a client during this time, or that she provide sexual services to her client in the same place. Clearly this will not always be possible. Another strategy was to ask another woman to note down the car number of the client, usually in full view of the client. This measure is used to deter men who might be contemplating any act which might involve violence. Noting down the car number, however, might not be sufficient to prevent trouble. It might, for example, be that the car is stolen, in which case the visible noting down of the number would be unlikely to act as a deterrent. Descriptive warnings about particular men are frequently circulated by word of mouth between women. These are generally taken seriously and heeded. However, as might be predicted with such informal communication networks, not everyone always hears such information.

Other strategies that street prostitutes use are to carry weapons or to have men in attendance while they work (usually boyfriends or husbands; Glasgow street prostitutes do not appear to have pimps). Neither of these strategies meets with police approval. The carrying of anything which might be used as a weapon can be legally construed as acting with intent to harm. As to the practice of having men in attendance, police are concerned to prevent any escalation of the tensions in the area as well as to limit the potential for activities such as drug dealing and muggings to occur. The reality for most prostitutes is that they work alone and if there is trouble with a client, there may well be no one else they can turn to for help at the time. This much said, there does appear to be a loose network of social support among Glasgow street prostitutes. At the least, this means that some women are prepared to respond actively to calls for help when women are being either verbally or physically assaulted by clients. This was demonstrated to us on a number of occasions where a woman's call for help met with an immediate response from nearby women. This raises the possibility of tapping into these networks and strengthening them for the purpose of making commercial sex safer for the collective of street prostitutes.

DESIGNING INTERVENTIONS

An enduring debate among policy makers and service providers has concerned the extent to which the target population should be involved in the design and implementation of strategies targeting risk behaviours. For the last few years the tide has run in favour of community-based peer-led interventions to change behaviour. The most prominent of these have been in relation to gay men, though such initiatives have been implemented with a wide variety of target groups (Rhodes, 1993). The underlying premise for these interventions is that there are unlikely to be many people better placed to contact the target population than members of that same population. They are also likely to be the best sources of information about the health needs of their community. One of the most impressive examples of using peer educators as credible sources of information has been the 'Gay Heroes' intervention employed in a number of US cities (see also Chapter 6). These programmes involve identifying highly regarded individuals within the local gay scene and recruiting them to act as peer educators to encourage a positive association with safer sex (Kelly et al., 1992). The existence of informal networks of mutual support among street prostitutes suggests the possibility that community-based interventions might be utilised to disseminate HIV prevention advice and more broadly defined safer sex messages, for example information regarding violent clients.

There are a number of good reasons for supposing that it is prostitutes themselves who are best placed to get across safer sex messages to other prostitutes. First, prostitutes have direct experience of negotiation with clients so they have a clearer sense of what is entailed in advocating behaviour change as well as an appreciation of the limits to what can be achieved (Wong et al., 1993). Second, it is important to have a credible source of information. This is perhaps more likely where the educator has direct experience of prostitution. Third, prostitutes may be better able than non-prostitutes to access certain areas used for commercial sex (Tchupo et al., 1993). Fourth, community-led interventions can encourage grass-roots activism and involvement. This implies a more dynamic approach to health education than is the case where issues are pre-defined and passed onto the community, often in the form of written information (Wiseman, 1988).

With adequate training and support, prostitutes could pass on their knowledge and experience to other prostitutes in ways which are seen to be appropriate and relevant. Prostitutes are often skilled negotiators, given that they are selling a service over which they see the need to retain a sense of control. However, these skills are unlikely to be uniformly distributed and there may well be marked differences in the negotiating styles of prostitutes. One study in Singapore found that some prostitutes were more successful than others in securing client compliance, in not succumbing to client pressure and in ensuring safer sex contacts (Wong et al., 1993). Having identified those prostitutes who were successful, these skills were then capitalised upon and used to try to improve the negotiation skills of women who were less able to secure client compliance. Self-evidently not all women will be suited to taking on the role of peer educator. This suggests the need to have a clearly defined understanding not only of what skills are needed but of how best to identify those women most able to convey and disseminate information. One possibility might be to target women who have a status analogous to that of the 'gay hero' (Kelly *et al.*, 1992) if such a role exists among street prostitutes.

A particularly valuable point of contact would be with women who have only recently begun to prostitute. Whilst many women are initiated into prostitution by women already working as prostitutes, this is not always the case. In the course of our research, we encountered approximately five women whose initiation into prostitution had been without advice or any kind of support. They had no pre-existing contacts with prostitutes prior to going to the red light district. Generally they knew nothing about dealing with clients, what to watch out for, how much money to charge and how to put a condom on a man even if they had condoms available. This is evident from the following field extract:

> One of the new women we encountered tonight had never worked as a prostitute before. She had approached one of the other women (Fiona) and appeared to be asking her about certain aspects of the job. She did not know Fiona. Fiona told the woman who we were, which saved her from getting any more anxious than she already looked. She had no condoms. I gave her some and explained which ones were for penetrative sex and which were for oral sex. In doing so I used the local term for oral sex (gams) which she didn't understand and laughed embarrassedly when I told her what it was. She was so obviously phased by the whole situation and was trying to psych herself up for her first encounter with a client. She asked Fiona to 'keep her right'. Fiona responded by laughing and shrugging off that responsibility saying 'I cannae even keep mysel' right, hen.'

Women such as this, with little or no understanding of what is involved in selling sex, have to be seen as extremely vulnerable. Assuming that the woman was clear about the use of prostitution as a source of income, contact with a peer educator at this point would have been valuable.

The mechanisms that might be used for disseminating information and skills amongst prostitute women would of course vary depending on the resources available. Prostitutes trained to act as peer educators could run workshops or educational sessions for other prostitutes, were premises available. They could take on the role of outreach workers combining peer education with the provision of condoms and, where appropriate, sterile injecting equipment. Whatever the mechanisms used, it appears that peer-led interventions are most likely to succeed where those involved feel they have ownership of the project, playing an active part in its creation, development and implementation (Pinzon, 1993; Cash and Anansuchatkul, 1993).

Much of what we have said so far may sound fine in theory, but one of the critical factors which would determine the success of any peer-led intervention is the question of whether there is in fact a community identity amongst women working as prostitutes.

ISSUES TO CONSIDER: A COMMUNITY OF INTEREST?

The blueprint for many community interventions is derived from HIV prevention work within the gay community. Although the notion of a gay community can itself be problematic, it is clear that there does exist a recognisable community of interest at both a social and a political level (Davies *et al.*, 1993). This cannot be assumed to be the case among injecting drug users (see Chapter 11) and prostitutes. Many prostitute women are working for the sole reason of funding an illegal and expensive drug habit, which in itself may militate against any long-lasting alliances. Among streetworking prostitutes the potential for collective response is also limited by the individualistic and competitive aspects of the work. Although we did come across women who worked in pairs and jointly pooled their money, such alliances were usually short-lived. For the most part women worked individually. It is unavoidable that prostitutes are to an extent in competition with each other. Such factors as the ratio of prostitutes to clients on any one night have an influence on how explicitly competitive the trade is. Another obvious intervening factor is the individual woman's need to earn money which might lead her to try to take another woman's client during the negotiation stage. Instances of this were often reported by the women and on several occasions also observed by us. Clearly the competitiveness implicit within street prostitution may cut across any simple notion that shared occupation equates with a sense of shared interest.

Furthermore, the shared experience of prostitution with its associated trials and tribulations is not enough to prevent some women from furthering their own ends by preying on others. So for example during our fieldwork we encountered one woman who was regularly extorting money from another prostitute and yet another who was mugging women for their earnings. This may be one reason why some women are distrustful or wary of other prostitutes and so for example avoid speaking much about the money they have earned:

> In commenting on how slow business seemed to be that night I asked Lara how much she'd managed to earn. She said £70 but added 'I'll tell you that, I'd of said one or two [clients] if anyone else asked or "I've no' done any."' She says she always underestimates if one of the other prostitutes asks her how much she's done.

A peer education project among male prostitutes in Brazil provides an example of the obstacles that may exist where the target population share little or nothing with each other beyond the fact of their involvement in selling sex. The work of the peer educators was obstructed by police harassment, by distrust and by competitiveness and hierarchy among male prostitutes. Peer educators were most successful in their own localities with male prostitutes with whom they had pre-existing social relations (Lorigo,1993).

Many gay men positively associate with the notion of a gay community. The same could not easily be said of many women who work as prostitutes, particularly on the streets. Clearly there are women who consider selling sex to be a job, and who are prepared to identify themselves as prostitutes and become actively involved in campaigning for prostitutes' rights. However, they are not in the majority. Many women shy away from identification as prostitutes because of the stigma attached to such work and its continuing social unacceptability (Darrow *et al.*, 1993). This lack of identification of a community of interest has consequences for the kinds of intervention which might be relevant or appropriate for streetworking prostitutes.

THE GREAT DIVIDE: INJECTORS AND NON-INJECTORS

Women prostitute to make money, but the reasons why they need the money may be more divisive than the mere fact of being involved in prostitution. In streetworking prostitution the most salient divide is usually between those women who are prostituting to finance a drug habit and those women who do not use drugs. In our own research a frequent source of tension amongst the women was the oft-voiced allegation by non-drug-injecting women that women who were injecting drugs were mugging clients, or providing sex without a condom, often for less than the accepted price. The following field extracts are illustrative of this:

> Lena was working up at the square which has been ruled out of bounds by the police. However, Lena says she prefers to take the risk and work there because 'there's nae fuckin' junkies, too many down the bottom and I hate 'em.' She says she doesn't use the drop-in centre for that reason and wishes that there were separate facilities for drug using prostitutes. She finished off saying, 'They're all out rippin' off punters for a start and doin' it for fivers [£5] and no' usin' [condoms].'

> We came across a group of women standing around a woman who had an infected abscess on her groin. She was lying on the floor in apparent agony. An ambulance had been called. One of the non-drug-using women came over to have a look. She [Elaine] can be quite aggressive and is very vocal in her disparagement of drug injecting. Seeing Tania on the floor she made some comment that it was all their own fault, to which one girl responded: 'You don't know what's it like when you've got a habit to feed.' Elaine then passed comment on another woman standing there [whom we know to be injecting drugs]. She feistily responded that she wasn't a junkie, that she didn't have a habit and that she had a wean [child]

to look after. Another woman turned to Elaine saying that she wasn't in a position to say anything anyway since she too was working as a prostitute. At this Elaine seemed to back down saying that she had a wean to look after too.

In recognition of the potential mistrust between drug using and non-drug-using women it seems important to recruit peer educators from both groups. Drug using prostitutes understand the additional pressures imposed by addiction and the effects this may have on working practices. Although any peer educator would need to be sensitive in approaching these issues, the scope for misunderstanding or antagonism might be less where the educator is also drug using and less likely to be cast as an accuser.

OWNERSHIP

Some evaluations of peer-led interventions have stressed the importance of ownership. A sense of ownership is said to increase where there is peer involvement in the project at all its stages. However, a related issue concerns payment and reward, particularly where the idea of community is weak. Prostitutes can generally earn sufficient money for their needs each night. Clearly the scope for earning money will be reduced during the times when they are acting as peer educators. The degree of ownership that prostitute peer educators feel may be closely related to the degree to which they feel they are rewarded, financially or otherwise. This may have particular resonance for women who are prostituting to finance a drug habit, whether their own or that of their partner.

INTERVENTIONS, SOCIAL SUPPORT AND INSTITUTIONAL BACK-UP

Interventions which are reliant on the skills and motivations of prostitutes will need to pay close attention to issues of recruitment, training and the provision of adequate support and back-up. Drug injecting prostitutes who act as peer educators may need particular support in recognition of their drug habit and the specific stresses this places on their lives. Friedman and colleagues have noted the need for pragmatism in work which draws on the resources of drug injectors to organise against HIV and AIDS (Friedman *et al.*,1992). Drug injectors' lives are often chaotic and unpredictable. The use of drug injecting prostitutes as peer educators would have to take cognisance of this and find a means of accommodating it.

Beyond using the skills extant within prostitution there are other means of trying to reduce the potential for unsafe or dangerous commercial sexual encounters. To an extent their success relies upon there being premises where prostitutes can meet during their working hours. One practical means of capitalising on prostitutes' experience and knowledge about troublesome or potentially violent clients is to have descriptions of such men on display in places where prostitutes meet (Morgan Thomas, 1992; McIver, 1992). Although police and prostitutes might appear to pull in opposing directions, given the laws regulating soliciting, some agencies have been able to develop good relations with police. It is one thing for women to take heed of warnings about particular men but it is also important to have sufficiently good relations with police for that information to be passed onto them. Where prostitutes have been attacked, it would be preferable for an assigned policewoman to come to the prostitute centre to take a statement if the woman wants to report it as a crime.

The development of good relations between police and prostitute service providers is an essential first step if women are to be encouraged to report such crimes. In particular, prostitutes have to feel confident that their allegations will be taken seriously. There is a view, probably shared by some police, that such women cannot be raped because of the nature of their work (Pheterson, 1988; Delacoste and Alexander, 1988). Indeed, some working women may have such a poor self-image that they have come to accept violence directed at themselves. Notions such as these discourage women from reporting rape or attack to the police. It is up to services and police to create the conditions where prostitutes feel it is worth their while reporting crimes against them. This begs the question of what happens once allegations against men come to court. Prostitutes have to confront the stigma of being labelled a common prostitute and the likely scepticism attaching to their credibility as victims. These factors dissuade many women from reporting violent assault by clients.

Health-related or social responses to prostitution are never far removed from the political domain, since so much of what happens in commercial sex is influenced by current legislation and public opinion. Most, if not all, of the measures which might be implemented to protect prostitutes are constrained by the illegalities surrounding commercial sex. The furtive and clandestine nature of the commercial sexual encounter created by legal and moral responses to prostitution actively increases the dangers streetworking prostitutes face. Decriminalisation would at least allow policy providers to consider measures for making commercial sex safer from both a public and an occupational health point of view. The decriminalisation of certain streets in Utrecht, the Netherlands, has resulted in the provision of purpose-built car parks for use by prostitutes and clients. These are well-lit, individually screened-off spaces where prostitutes can provide sexual services in a relatively safe environment (Kleinegris, 1991). Such measures in Britain would be thwarted by the law and very possibly by public opposition. However, it is worth pointing out that the provision of prostitute drop-in facilities stands somewhat in opposition to the legal status to prostitution. Nonetheless, a compelling case for their implementation has been successfully made in many British cities.

The new pragmatism which has allowed the provision of facilities in response to concerns about HIV spread has not extended to ensuring a safer working environment for prostitute women. At least part of this reluctance is rooted in deep-seated social prejudices against prostitutes and prostitution. These justify our concerns that prostitutes might act as vectors for disease but prevent us from considering the health and other needs that prostitutes themselves might have. The impetus provided by HIV prevention has been to contact prostitutes and go some way towards recognising the realities of streetworking prostitution. Services targeted at prostitutes, whether peer-led or not, need to go beyond HIV. We have an opportunity to build on and improve the services delivered to a marginalised and stigmatised group. Irrespective of our personal views on whether the legal status of prostitution should be changed, we should take that opportunity.

NOTE

The Centre for Drug Misuse Research is funded by the Chief Scientist Office of the Scottish Home and Health Department. The opinions expressed in this chapter are not necessarily those of the Scottish Home and Health Department.

REFERENCES

Barnard, M.A. (1992) 'Working in the dark: researching female prostitution', in H. Roberts (ed.) *Women's Health Matters*, London: Routledge.

Barnard, M.A. (1993) 'Violence and vulnerability: conditions of work for street-working prostitutes', *Sociology of Health and Illness*, 15: 683–705.

Bloor, M., Barnard, M.A., Finlay, A. and McKeganey, N. (1993) 'HIV-related risk practices among Glasgow male prostitutes: reframing concepts of risk behaviour', *Medical Anthropology Quarterly*, 7: 152–69.

Carr, S., Green, S., Goldberg, D., Cameron, S., Gruer, L., Frischer, M., Mackie, T. and Follet, E. (1992) 'HIV prevalence among female street prostitutes attending a health-care drop-in centre in Glasgow', *AIDS*, 6: 1553–54.

Cash, K. and Anansuchatkul, B. (1993) 'Relevant AIDS education for Thai adolescent female workers', IX International Conference on AIDS, Berlin (Abstract, WS–D04–3).

Darrow, W., Potterat, J., Alegria, N., Rios, M. and Woodhouse, D. (1993) 'HIV prevention for streetwalkers: are condoms enough?' IX International Conference on AIDS, Berlin (Abstract, WS–CO8–5).

Davies, P., Hickson, F., Weatherburn, P. and Hunt, A. (1993) *Sex, Gay Men and AIDS*, Brighton: Falmer Press.

Delacoste, F. and Alexander, P. (1988) *Sex Work: Writings by Women in the Sex Industry*, London: Virago Press.

Friedman, S., Sufian, M., Curtis, R., Neaigus, A. and Des Jarlais, D. (1992) 'Organising drug users against AIDS', in J. Huber and B. Schneider (eds) *The Social Context of AIDS*, London: Sage.

Hepburn, M. (1992) 'Pregnancy and HIV: screening, counselling and services', in J. Bury, V. Morrison and S. McLachlan (eds) *Working with Women and AIDS: Medical, Social and Counselling Issues*, London: Routledge.

Kelly, J., St Lawrence, J., Stevenson, Y., Hauth, A., Kalichman, S., Diaz, Y., Brasfield, T., Koob, J. and Morgan, M. (1992) 'Community AIDS/HIV risk reduction: the effects of endorsements by popular people in three cities', *American Journal of Public Health*, 82: 1483–89.

Kleinegris, M. (1991) 'Innovative AIDS prevention among drug-using prostitutes'. Paper presented at Second International Conference on the Reduction of Drug-Realted Harm, Barcelona.

Lorigo, P. (1993) 'A larger concept of peer education: the experience of Programa "Pegacao"'. IX International Conference on AIDS, Berlin (Abstract, WS–D10–6).

McIver, N. (1992) 'Developing a service for prostitutes in Glasgow', in J. Bury, V. Morrison and S. McLachlan (eds) *Working with Women and AIDS: Medical, Social and Counselling Issues*, London: Routledge.

McKeganey, N. and Barnard, M.A. (1992) 'Selling sex: female street prostitution and HIV risk behaviour in Glasgow', *AIDS Care*, 4,4: 395–407.

McKeganey, N., Barnard, M.A., Leyland, A., Coote, I. and Follet, E. (1992) 'Female streetworking prostitution and HIV infection in Glasgow', *British Medical Journal*, 305: 801–4.

McKeganey, N.P., Barnard, M.A. and Bloor, M.J. (1993) 'Estimating prostitute numbers: epidemiology out of ethnography', in M. Boulton (ed.) *Methodological Advances in Behavioural Research on AIDS*, Brighton: Falmer Press.

Matthews, L. (1990) 'Outreach work with female prostitutes in Liverpool', in M. Plant (ed.) *AIDS, Drugs and Prostitution*, London: Routledge.

Morgan Thomas, R. (1992) 'HIV and the sex industry', in J. Bury, V. Morrison and S. McLachlan (eds) *Working with Women and AIDS: Medical, Social and Counselling Issues*, London: Routledge.

Pheterson, G. (1988) 'The social consequences of unchastity', in F. Delacoste and P. Alexander (eds) *Sex Work: Writings by Women in the Sex Industry*, London: Virago Press.

Pinzon, A. (1993) 'Combining alternative communication and participatory processes as a form of peer education', IX International Conference on AIDS, Berlin (Abstract, WS–D13–5).

Rhodes, T. (1993) 'Time for community change: what has outreach to offer?', *Addiction*, 88: 1317–20.

Shedlin, M. (1990) 'An ethnographic approach to understanding HIV high-risk behaviours: prostitution and drug abuse', in C. Lenkefeld, R. Battjes and Z. Amsel (eds) *AIDS and Intravenous Drug Use: Community Interventions and Prevention*, New York: Hemisphere Publishing Corporation.

Silbert, M. (1981) *Sexual Assault of Prostitutes*, San Francisco: Delaney Street Foundation.

Synn Stern, L. (1992) 'Self-injection education for street level sex workers', in P. O'Hare, R. Newcombe, A. Matthews, E. Buning and E. Drucker (eds) *The Reduction of Drug-Related Harm*, London: Routledge.

Tchupo, J., Manchester, T., Monny Lobe, M. and Buschel, R. (1993) 'The importance of peer distribution of condoms to prostitutes', IX International Conference on AIDS, Berlin (Abstract, WS–D10–4).

Ward, H., Day, S., Mezzone, J., Dunlop, L., Donegan, C., Farrar, S., Whitaker, L., Harris, J. and Miller, D. (1993) 'Prostitution and risk of HIV: female prostitutes in London', *Brithish Medical Journal*, 307: 356–58.

Wiseman, T. (1988) 'Marginalised groups and health education about HIV infection and AIDS', in P. Aggleton, G. Hart and P. Davies (eds) *AIDS: Social Representations, Social Practices*, Brighton: Falmer Press.

Wong, M., Archibald, C., Roy, K., Chan, C., Goh, A., Goh, C. and Tan, T. (1993) 'A qualitative investigation of condom use negotiation among prostitutes in Singapore', IX International Conference on AIDS, Berlin (Abstract, WS–D10–1).

Chapter 8

Save sex/save lives*

Evolving modes of activism

Cindy Patton

The prerogative to apply names is one of the most contentious forms of power in the late twentieth century. Disenfranchised groups had high hopes for the names and concepts they forged for themselves in the 1960s and 1970s. But the 1980s and 1990s have been a sobering object lesson in the relatively greater power held by science, government, and media to name, rename, and take over the names groups make for themselves. AIDS organisers and activists learned a hard lesson: it is difficult to predict results of discursive battles. But this is not just a problem of securing activists' *meanings*. Ideas proposed by activists are taken up and modified by officials, rendering activism partially successful, but without affording activists any real power.

Many view ACT UP's New York début in 1987 as the beginning of activism, perhaps including 'grass roots' projects by sex workers or 'self-help' groups formed by people living with AIDS as proto-activisms.[1] This view counts only the most publicly oppositional work as 'activist': demonstrations, angry proclamations, symbolic hand grenades thrown from a position of extreme exclusion from 'the system'. But even by this traditional definition, ACT UP did not remain totally oppositional for long. By 1989, the organising committees of AIDS conferences were meeting with ACT UP chapters in advance, and by 1992, ACT UP's 'actions' at the Amsterdam International Aids conference were run according to a schedule, partially negotiated with conference organisers, to minimise disruption and maximise press coverage. This is less a comment on ACT UP's ability to sustain a fully oppositional posture – indeed, they do not themselves hold to this traditional definition – than emblematic of the form that activist politics now takes, at least in the HIV epidemic. Increasingly, radical critique is not so much 'telling it like it is' in order to rip the scales of ideology from people's eyes as it is complexly enmeshed in the process of constructing and reconstructing discursive and institutional power.

The naming of the epidemic provides an easy example of the dynamics of this process. 'AIDS' maintained its ideological connection with Western gay men through three changes in nomenclature – Gay Related Immune Deficiency (GRID), Acquired Immune Deficiency Syndrome (AIDS), Human Immunodeficiency Virus (HIV) disease – which reflected different understandings of the relation between bodies and disease. Activists' accusations of homophobia, along with the scientific recognition that there were many cases among people other than gay men, prompted the change from GRID to AIDS. Activists then critiqued use of the probably fatal late stage of a longer, chronic viral process as the name for the complex as a whole. The connotative value of AIDS as a 'death sentence' was seen as fatalistic and psychologically harmful to those who had the virus (Callen, 1988). Many scientists agreed, but for reasons of their own: a term like 'HIV spectrum' or 'HIV disease' better reflected the course of the virus and the varying levels of medical intervention which those who had it might wish to entertain (see Centers for Disease Control [CDC], 1986; Redfield *et al.*, 1986).[2]

But despite these interventions and changes, the AIDS–gay connection held fast. The activist–scientist struggle over names was only the most superficial level of a whole range of namings which stemmed from the deep – and continuing – association of the medical phenomenon with a group of people thought to have a unique trait which makes them deviant. 'GRID' suggests that pathology resulted from something 'gay-related': here, the syndrome and those who have it are synonymous. But 'AIDS' taps another complex cultural discourse: 'choosing' to be 'gay' is easily equated with 'acquiring' 'immunodeficiency'. Even the 'spectrum' of 'HIV disease' tracks a cultural trope: both Freudian views of sexuality and Queer Nation's explosion of narrow ideas of gay identity suggest that most people are more or less queer. But instead of exploding homophobia, notions of polymorphous perversity fed the belief that those who could secure their heterosexuality would not contract the slow-acting virus.

The AIDS–gay association which has shaped activism, policy, representation, and research is more than a tragic example of deeply entrenched homophobia. In fact, a whole range of ideas – challenged and enlisted by activists – stem from this early codification. It is critical that activists in the 1990s understand that the challenges they pose are partially contingent on ideas that grew out of the interaction of the initial, blatantly homophobic conceptions of the disease with activists' responses to it.[3] These central, virtually naturalised ideas are now embedded in policy and representational logics, sometimes serving as a lever for activism, but sometimes splitting activists along gender and racial lines.

In particular, I want to argue here, the connotations of 'identity' and 'community' which related these terms to urban gay men's experience and activism are central terms through which the epidemic is understood. This partial incorporation of gay men's ideas of themselves into the research/ policy/media enterprise has resulted in a significant loss of control over the terms used to stage activism. Not only has this created problems among gay male activists (How to deal with 'men who have sex with men'? Nudge them toward 'gay identity' or be 'culturally sensitive' and let them practice *ex nominatio*), but it has affected organising efforts across the categories naturalised by epidemiology: between gay men and women, and between gay men and people of colour.

Weaving together political history and an evaluation of health education strategies, I will take my own experiences in a range of safe-sex organising projects through the 1980s in the US as the central example in this chapter. Growing out of a huge, market-based health care system and highly decentralised research, public health, and media systems, the US case is arguably unique. However, activist safe-sex projects and ACT UP have been cloned in many parts of the Western world. Perhaps more importantly, as the major centre for naming and directing the policy and research course of the epidemic, the activist–official struggle within the US strongly influences the general landscape of policy and discourse far beyond the nation's borders. Hopefully, readers will forgive my parochialism; my discussion is intended to form a historical backdrop for raising questions about local activism in the US and elsewhere, as well as suggesting some of the sources of international conflicts over activists' strategies.

This chapter will suggest that particular notions of 'community' and 'identity' were consolidated through active efforts on the part of gay men to reorganise their collective sexual practice. This occurred in the context of a more diffuse and contradictory series of representations of 'safe sex' to and sometimes for the 'general public'. While I hope that re-evaluation of these interactions proves useful to discussions of activism in the 1990s, there can be no ultimate resolution of the tension between the 'mainstream' and 'community' understandings of 'safe sex', since official naming bodies – media, government agencies, research and policy enterprises – finally have more power to disperse meanings.

THE SHIFTING POLITICS OF SEX EDUCATION

Even before the term 'safe sex' was coined, gay men had begun to organise to avoid 'acquiring' the hazily understood new disease. While drawing on some traditional health education models, this early work – some five years before ACT UP formed – entailed crucial activist intervention at a time of official silence about the epidemic. Important and formative battles about sexuality were waged on three fronts in these early years of resistance: to get sex spoken of publicly, to get researchers to understand the nuance and detail of gay men's sexual practices, and to dissociate specific practices from the broader 'gay identity' which had been of critical political significance for gay men and lesbians as they articulated themselves as a minority in order to achieve civil rights.[4]

Ironically, through extensive debate and involvement in early epidemiologic study, men who claimed 'gay identities' were partially successful at dislinking identity from sexual acts. This meant that research could focus on specific, clear *routes* of transmission while allowing that gay *sexuality* included many activities that were always 'safe'. The strength of gay men's response also made it clear that there *were* gay communities, many of which also included lesbians and other people whose sexualities did not fit comfortably within the mainstream. These collective responses afforded organised gay communities (primarily in the northern European countries, the US, Canada, and Australia) some power in shaping policy.

Both identity and community originally had strong connotative meanings: identity was largely oppositional ('not straight') and community marked subcultural affinity. But the media still collapsed identity and practices, and 'heterosexuality' was commonly transformed into a default identity (Patton, 1985b). Men with a gay identity were all presumed to engage in specific 'risky' homosexual acts, but the absence of those acts in others conveyed to them a heterosexual identity. Similarly, community was confused with 'risk group': the gay community in general was popularly considered to be 'at risk', and not from homophobia, as activists argued, but from their sexuality.

Once it became clear that 'anyone can get AIDS', this confusion provided a corollary 'safe' space for non-gay people. By the end of the 1980s, researchers and the media would frequently replace the word 'mainstream' with the phrase 'heterosexual community' to indicate those non-gay, sexually active people who might be at risk of contracting HIV. But a 'heterosexual community' was a simulacrum produced by epidemiology and the media. It lacked the social reality of the 'gay community', which, through decades of defending members against homophobia, had forged a social geography, produced common interests and values, and consolidated resources like alternative media, businesses, and clinics.

FROM COMMUNITY RESISTANCE TO 'SAFE SEX': 1981–86

The first safe-sex projects were conceptualised during the initial early period of extreme scientific uncertainty. Early AIDS activists had to fight against indifference *while* the researchers and clinicians settled on their own scientific logic. Not only did scientists not agree on the general progression of the new syndrome, but they did not even agree on its cause. Some believed that there must be an aetiologic agent which was most likely sexually transmissible. However, many others viewed the 'gay lifestyle' as the cause: use of drugs, perhaps even auto-immune response to semen were hypothesised to result in the observed immune system failure. Because of this lack of consensus, 'advice' developed by activists had to cover a lot of ground. The initial broad-stroke approach to theories of AIDS aetiology, reversed in the later overemphasis on transmission of HIV alone, strongly influenced how risk reduction advice to gay men was framed.

This was an excruciatingly uncertain time for early organisers: the number of men with 'prodromal' symptoms who were projected to progress to AIDS

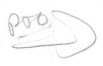

increased almost weekly, from 5 per cent to 10 per cent to 100 per cent, even as projected life span from diagnosis got longer. Activists knew they needed to disrupt transmission (if, indeed, there was a transmissible agent) or rebuild immune systems, but they also needed to help scientists gain insight into the syndrome's 'natural history'. In the absence of computer models, scientists were tempted to withdraw from intervening. Gay men absolutely demanded that any epidemiologic study include serious and aggressive promotion of risk reduction, even if this introduced a virtually unmeasurable variable which turned descriptive studies of the *epidemic* into evaluation studies of educational strategies. Scientists would ultimately comply, but would again raise the issue of 'natural history' versus intervention regarding AZT trials.[5] They would scour the globe in search of groups who could be argued to be intransigent to advice – because they were illiterate, forced into prostitution by poverty, or because their sex drive was considered unamenable to change.

Even before 1984, when HIV was identified as the probable (though we now know, not sufficient) cause of immune system breakdown, major efforts were under way within the US gay communities to promote sexual precautions. By about 1986, the myriad approaches to prevention were consolidated under the name 'safe', and later, 'safer sex'. It is hard to remember what it was like to organise for risk reduction with no single covering term; the title of the Callen–Berkowitz manual, *How to Have Sex in an Epidemic* (1983) recalls the time. But soon the idea of safe or safer sex implicitly collaborated with the idea that queer sex was in itself unsafe. In the context of bifurcated 'communities' – gay versus mainstream/heterosexual – queer sex had to be *made* safe while heterosexual sex was safe until queered.

Few risk reduction or health education efforts emerged from the official US public health offices until 1986, when it appeared that heterosexuals could become infected with HIV, converting the 'public' into a 'community'. From 1986 to the present, education efforts for and by gay men have faced clear limits due to the Helms Amendment.[6] But the limitations on safe-sex education were not caused by direct censorship alone: both the Helms Amendment and traditional health education theory shared the premise that homosexuality could be neatly defined, and the homosexual easily flushed out. Both assumed that homosexuals uniformly experience and recognise – or could be educated to recognise – their sexual condition. The idea that sexual activities equal social identity (i.e. same-sex acts lead to gay identity) and that any mismatch between acts and identity was a result of misrecognition or repression also characterised much of the safe-sex educational effort coming from within gay communities.

Uncritically adopting general concepts from health education, the first risk reduction efforts within the US gay community, from 1981 to 1983, used straightforward information to identify and change the sexual and drug use behaviours believed to be related to AIDS. Early campaigns included advice about changing aspects of 'lifestyle' which we now know may affect progression of HIV illness but have nothing to do with initial infection. These campaigns of 'don'ts' (or 'don't until'), coming from within the gay community and its clinics, were criticised by other gay people as sexually repressive. These new 'activists', who saw themselves as opposing gay groups that had grown too close to the official voices, viewed advice against anal intercourse as intrinsically homophobic, but gay activists internationally disagreed about whether condoms were safe enough, especially in light of the growing awareness that science would have no quick means of eliminating HIV and that change would be for the long haul.

These first campaigns also failed to recognise that sexual acts and the language used to describe and enact them already carried a surplus of meanings. Activists argued that the term 'promiscuity' was inaccurate and that 'anonymous sex' had been misunderstood by researchers. The advice to decrease and to know one's partners negatively interpreted gay male socio-sexual organisation, overemphasising total reported partners and fantasising risk in dangerous places instead of in specific acts. You don't need to 'know' your partner to engage in transmission-disrupting acts, activists argued, and the statistical odds of avoiding HIV by decreasing the number of partners alone only worked if the pool of potential partners was itself low in seroprevalence. If seroprevalence rates were 50 or 60 or 80 per cent, as reported in some tightly-knit groups in urban gay ghettos or among drug users or among men with haemophilia A who had received Factor VIII before 1985, then reducing numbers did little to reduce statistical risk.

Many individual men changed their sexual practices during these confusing early years, but these changes were often overwhelmed by changes in the structure and ethos of gay male communities: survivor's guilt, loss of friends and the stress of coping with the health crisis and accompanying political backlash competed with efforts to recognise and celebrate gay men's collective bid for survival through safe sex. Gay men experienced a loss of identity because the acts viewed as problematic were, for some men, simply 'what gay men do'. In addition, the possibility of drawing many partners, from a wide range of venues with different symbolic–erotic structures, had created a large network of sexual and relationship options for many gay men. The places they had forged as safe havens for meeting other men (bars, bathhouses, public parks, porn cinemas, the fresh-fruit aisle of the Star Market) were now recast as dangerous places, populated by dangerous men. For many, the suggestion to reduce the number of partners and the vilification of particular venues that once symbolised the gains of gay subculture in articulating a collective safe space (especially bathhouses and backroom bars) felt like a loss of community.

A second phase of gay-community-controlled, activist 'education', from about 1983 to 1986, tried to correct the negativity of initial efforts which seemed to have produced despair, incredulity, or uncertainty. But these efforts were complicated by new science and shifting ideas about the epidemic. Until this time, epidemiologists, activists, and those concerned about their health had focused on 'the past' – how did AIDS start? What historical strengths in our community can we draw on? Did *I* do anything 'dangerous' in the late 1970s? The discovery of a virus created a future. Demographers and epidemiologists began to develop computer models to simulate the epidemic. The information presented in the media and at AIDS conferences (widely attended by early activists – not to protest, but to infiltrate the central place where one acquired a degree in 'AIDSology') suggested that gay men's future looked bleak: safe-sex education could no longer be viewed as an interim set of measures until medicine put things right.

The stopgap view of safe sex was problematic for several reasons: it proposed the wrong motive and strategy for change – something like giving up certain foods until a weight loss goal is reached. The stopgap approach was grounded in scare tactics and proposed an explanation for why some people didn't change: either they were fatalistic or sexually compulsive. The stopgap approach blamed the social backlash accompanying AIDS on social anxieties about AIDS, indicting AIDS phobia – rooted in ignorance – rather than indicting the persistent homophobia that was enacted through queer-bashing, or more diffusely, through individual intolerance that lent support to continued systematic discrimination against gay people (and, perhaps even more consistently and coherently, against prostitutes). In addition, the new focus on a single virus narrowed discussion of prevention to the disruption of HIV transmission only, initially disregarding potentially transmissible co-factors and discounting the more general immune system enhancing 'life-style' choices which would prove crucial in slowing progression of symptoms and improving quality of life for those infected.

The vast media coverage suggesting that HIV would be around for decades reframed safe-sex advice. In the already widening gulf between advice to gay men and advice to heterosexuals, gay men were required to make radical changes but no general social revolution in sexual–technical norms was required. With the tide of increasing moral conservatism, calls to sexual austerity quickly overran calls for heterosexuals also to take up condoms as a universal precaution. The question was no longer how but whether to have sex: the 'sexual revolution' was over. But while key gay ghettos saw a levelling of new seroconversions among adult men by the mid- to late 1980s, it was unclear that 'waiting' (increasing age of onset of intercourse) or 'faithfulness' (decrease in number of partners) among younger people in similarly high prevalence areas would forestall new 'waves' of infection. The failure to advocate condoms as a cultural norm meant that when youths had sex, they did it without condoms – 'the real thing' was the reward for waiting and for being faithful (at least, on a serial basis). Indeed, HIV infections among the young in cities where HIV was well-established skyrocketed in the late 1980s and through to the present.[7]

HISTORY AND RESISTANCE

As the idea of a 'heterosexual community' took hold, the oppositional form and historical place of gay community began to fade from view, especially for younger gay people who must now have seen 'community' as a neutral descriptor for two 'lifestyle' 'choices'. The analysis of the sources of oppression shifted the nature and project of community organising as it had first emerged in relation to AIDS and risk reduction. Energy went into re-educating the public, not about gay life, but about how you 'can't get AIDS from a doorknob'. Instead of helping individuals recognise their own relationship to and possible membership of the gay community, instead of describing the fluidity of sexuality, or preserving recent gay history, educators conveyed technical information about viruses and condom efficacy. Young men who entered gay worlds in the 1980s often seemed to interpret gay liberation as a simple, selfish libertinism, a cause of AIDS. The displacement of the responsibility for the effects of homophobia onto gay culture or gay liberation undermined the strength and values which gay communities had honed over decades of resisting social repression. Safe sex was now understood as the effect for which libertinism was the cause: taken out of the context of a history of homosexuality and its repression, the imposition of safe sex became a punishment for someone else's misdeeds. In a history of resistance against queer-bashing, psychological terrorism (lobotomy, aversion therapy, institutionalisation), medical indifference (untreated sexually transmitted diseases, no research on special health needs, no preventative or primary care), police harassment, job and housing discrimination, and ridicule, safe sex might have been interpreted as another form of fighting back. But without the collective memory of earlier forms of homosexual repression, safe sex reopened parts of the gay community to the same kinds of psychological and social policing which were at the heart of the government's failure to respond to the HIV epidemic in the first place. Instead of understanding changing norms as an intra-community project, warring groups of gay men blamed each other for stretching the boundaries of sexual experimentation.

Though conflicting and contentious, safe-sex campaigns within gay communities probably contributed in some way to changing individual behaviour. However, their long-term effect has been to help shore up the split between 'normal' and 'deviant' sex, bringing the latter further into the reach of the long arm of the state. Gay men's and sex workers' expression of their sexuality are now barely separable from the descriptions and survey categories of state epidemiology. Although they vary in gay-positiveness and capacity to enable resistance to social oppression, few existing projects directly challenge the policing of sexuality. While it is impossible to separate the effects of any one project or approach from the broader social-change process, it is possible to describe the general trajectory of safe-sex projects.

INFORMATION MODEL

In crude terms, the information model locates the unhealthy behaviour in the individual and explains behaviour as an effect of ignorance. The solution is information. The model makes two assumptions: first, that among ordinary people, information will change attitudes and awareness, which will induce a desire to change, which will eventually result in change. Second, this normal progression breaks down: the educated person either shows no desire to change or is unsuccessful at making a desired change. These individuals are viewed as recalcitrant or compulsive, refusing to accept the consequences of their behaviour or unable to control the drive toward their negative behaviour.

A major problem of the information model is its self-perpetuating claim about knowledge: as long as information is seen as effective in itself, rather than only the most preliminary beginning, lack of behaviour change will suggest that not enough or the wrong information has been provided. Information campaigns begets information campaigns, and social science evaluation of them begets more research. The complexity of administering such a volume of information stabilises health education institutions, which then have financial and political commitments to sustaining information campaigns and their evaluation. But worse, it produces the illusion that risk reduction is highly complex and technical. Where most people once learned their sexual techniques from discussion with friends or in action with their partners, individuals now get the impression that they need extensive and professional assistance to sort through the menu of safe sex practices.

Finally, the assumptions of the information model, now crystallised in health education institutions, set a limit on government and social responsibility for promoting sexual health. At some point, those who fail to respond to information are declared 'hard to reach'. To the extent that people so designated happen to match up to pre-existing demographic units – African American and Latino youth, sex workers, bisexual men – society, through the long arm of public health policing, can declare them expendable by blaming the failure of misguided information campaigns on the traits stereotyped as characteristic of the group. The traditional information model, by denying the role of community norms, rationalises punitive actions against the very people the model has failed.

PSYCHOLOGICAL DEFICIT MODEL

Psychological deficit models are therapeutic solutions for those who have not responded to information campaigns due to their perceived inability to make an apparently rational change. Again, the problem is situated in the individual. The institutionally supported and grass roots groups which emerged in the mid-1980s to address 'sexual compulsiveness' in gay men were based in this model, but the fact that individuals perceive *themselves* to be 'compulsive' in no way validates the model. It should not be surprising that people who believe in the information model, but find themselves unable to accomplish the prescribed change, might come to believe that there was something wrong with themselves. Gay men struggle daily against a culture that believes they are pathological: when risk of HIV is equated in nearly every popular media outlet with number of partners and with homosexuality diffusely, what was once viewed as a healthy desire for sex is reinterpreted as a pathological desire for dangerous sex. Some gay men who found it hard to take up risk-reducing practices found a reasuring, quasi-medical explanation in the idea of their 'compulsiveness': groups promised to protect them from fatal desires that they could not control in themselves.

The 'Hot, Horny, and Healthy' workshop, designed by Michael Chernoff in New York City and used since the mid-1980s, was an important step away from projects that proposed abstinence in place of sexual activities now labelled compulsive or fatal. These workshops were probably most helpful during the years when men who had experienced a very different set of cultural norms sought to reorganise their sexuality. The workshops helped men reconstitute their sexuality through 'eroticising' safe practices in the context of perceived new values of mutual responsibility. While it remains one of the most significant educational models, 'Hot, Horny, and Healthy' makes several troubling assumptions which stemmed from the period in which they were designed. There is an uncomfortable assumption that sexuality must be tamed through mature and rational limit setting, to be effected through verbal 'communication' and 'intimacy'. The overemphasis on verbal communication misunderstands the role gestural, spatial, and symbolic modes play in shaping and changing situational norms. In these programmes safe sex is less a transmission-disrupting choreography of bodies than a coordinated discourse about them. In addition, it reconstitutes the 1970s as a mythical time in which 'anything went', rewriting the highly codified and ritualistic gay male culture of that time as lacking in norms and moral values.

Most complexly, while components of these programmes deal with non-penetrative sexual options, they ultimately situate intercourse as the real sex, even if only by invoking intercourse as that which is lost and must now be mourned. This tacitly reduces to poor substitute or foreplay the very practices which were once considered fetishistically absorbing and gratifying and are the safest practices from the standpoint of HIV transmission. This view of anal intercourse as especially identity-conveying is a significant change from the late 1970s ethos, when sexual specificity – transgression, fetishism – rather than intercourse *per se* was the source of oppositional gay identity. This cultural shift in what constitutes real gay sex precariously and dangerously rearticulates gay male sexuality to, and defines gay identity in terms of, the one act it has had to modify. In a sense, the new social definition of gayness as merely different by choosing intercourse with men rather than women narrowed male identity – gay or straight – by staking it on performance of the most transmission-enabling practice. Gay sex was not only heterosexualised, it was made fatal by definition: avoiding intercourse altogether made one *safe* but not really gay, not really heterosexual, not really a *man*.

With its heterosexist and Victorian unconscious, safe sex practice was now overdetermined by its role in demarcating transgressive sex from mature or safe sex. For men who continued to view gay sex as intrinsically transgressive of cultural or individual psychic norms, the loss of transgressiveness which safe sex implies eliminated a critical component of their desires.

COMMUNITY DEFICIT PROGRAMMES

The widely used Stop AIDS project was the first major move away from individual or group work-oriented programmes. In its initial form, Stop AIDS utilised the pedagogic theories of Paolo Freire (1973). These employ a diffusion model which assumes that social change occurs because a small number of well-informed and motivated individuals effect changes through their interaction with a larger number of people. The model organised a vanguard to speed up cultural change; when a critical mass had been reached, the project ended and community change continued on its course. The programme held meetings and made individual contacts with the goal of advocating safe sex as a community organising project. The meetings promoted community solidarity and provided basic safe-sex information. Although these programmes had high visibility and boasted large numbers of individual contacts, Stop AIDS did not adequately assess how sexual norms are established, changed, and maintained in specific urban gay communities. It attempted to promote normative change in group settings separate from the situations and social spaces in which sex was enacted. Unlike the paradigmatic Freirean literacy projects, Stop AIDS misunderstood that while critical reading skills may be acquired, possessed, and carried around, 'sexual literacy' does not easily translate from space to space. No does not reliably mean no, and practitioners vary their enforcement of their own rules depending on their partner and their specific, temporally and spatially situated erotic goal. Stop AIDS turned out to be more like Alcoholics Anonymous than Freire's literacy programmes in that it created a separate space for reflection on the hazards of sex, rather than transforming the places in which sex occurs into ones supportive of safe-sex norms. And because it closed its doors at some point, Stop AIDS did not even provide this ongoing safe space and lost its capacity to directly challenge evolving sexual norms from within the spaces where problematic sexual practices were believed to occur.

COMMUNITY EMANCIPATION MODEL

By the late 1980s, several cities (Austin, Texas; Sydney, New South Wales; Boston, Massachusetts) and ACT UP in a variety of cities, decided to improve on the Stop AIDS concept, moving toward community organising projects grounded quite overtly in *gay* liberation and social construction theory. These projects understood the practice of sex to be highly site-specific and particip-ants to be widely different in their identities and motivations, requiring organisers to work differently in a wide variety of venues. These projects viewed pre-epidemic gay male culture as highly organised, with strong and easily understood norms supportive of community formation and the pro-duction of individual gay identities. The projects rejected the idea that the epidemic required a radical break from the sexual ideology of the recent past, and rejected moves to vilify or idealise the 1970s as a time of individual sexual licence and community adolescence which needed to be replaced by individual and group maturity.

The emancipatory model challenged the 'that was then, this is now' ethos of most other projects by celebrating the continuity and usefulness of sexual styles and negotiation patterns from the 1970s to the 1980s. The perception that 1970s gay culture was chaotic and normless was viewed as self-defeating and as incorrectly based on the premise that sex is a drive which tends toward specific goals and that had now to be diverted. Instead, sexuality was understood as constantly in the process of construction and resymbolisation. The inarticulateness of 1970s gay norms postulated by early programmes (belied by the sheer volume of books, travel guides, and folklore about how and where to pick up men) was the result of the naturalisation of community practices; gay male culture was not normless, but had integrated norms so well that they were no longer consciously perceived. The norms of the 1970s may not have been recognisable as 'communication', and were frequently not 'intimate', but the system of semiotic codes and venue specificities was reliable. In a short time, an individual could follow the migrations and changes in style which gay sex employed to avoid policing and easily find types of sex or styles of men at particular bars or in particular places. Seeking sex and seeking relationships were largely two different enterprises, often accomplished by using different strategies and different locations. These emancipatory projects took pains to incorporate memories of resistance and celebration from the recent gay past: they shared an assumption that community norms change more quickly when men identify old rules as a positive process to be adapted rather than perceiving themselves to be isolated individuals moving from an unrestricted culture into one now rife with rules which one must learn as a novice.

As in Freire's projects, participants in these projects began with critical exploration of the meaning and rules of their own specific sexual worlds. They made conscious the norms and problems they confronted and solved daily. In this context, safe sex was viewed as a norm in process, not a problem. These projects promoted positive attitudes toward gay male sexuality and included safe sex practice as part of what makes gay sexuality an important bond for community; a culture that supports gay male sexuality will support evolving changes in behaviour and norms. Thus, safe sex was viewed as part of the larger and ongoing project of sexual liberation, organising for which did not end when a specific behaviour change had been accomplished. Although achieving specific changes in behavioural norms was urgent and imperative, the larger goal was promoting community processes that increased the resilience of gay male culture as a whole. On the individual and community levels, working to make sex safe was an act of resistance to a homophobic culture. Safe-sex organising worked closely with HIV/AIDS support and gay liberation projects as forms of community building rather than being a separate and individualistic campaign for personal change.

SAFE SEX WITHOUT IDENTITY, SAVE SEX OUTSIDE COMMUNITY

Changing same-sex sexual norms requires strengthening the communities and *situations* of the practitioners of homosexuality. Emancipatory projects recognised the hazards of an overly narrow concept of sexual community, since many, perhaps even most, practitioners of same-sex relations do not identify as gay. There has been considerable debate about the value of promoting gay identity, but there is still not a solid case for comprehensive promotion of the urban-core-type gay identity. Activists are now moving away from organising around identity and community and are thinking more specifically about venues and forms of homosexual practices.

The historical reality is that gay identity as we know it formed most visibly around white middle-class forms of same-sex relations. These are the figures of gay men and lesbians promoted in the media, by politicians (including 'our own') and as epidemiology. People of colour and men and women from other cultures and classes in which bisexuality is an unspoken norm are in jeopardy if 'community' demands narrow self-identification with the white middle-class 'coming out' developmental ideology of the past two decades of gay liberation. All sexual spaces and forms have their rules of emergence and of practice, whether or not those who enter into them consider themselves to 'be' gay. Safe-sex organisers must support these unnamed sexual networks as well as the larger, self-named gay community if we are to effectively resist the increased social control over sexuality which jeopardises safe sex and its incorporation into our cultures.

I do not believe that creating a resistance movement capable of making sex safe (from disease and social repression) requires recruiting everyone to gay identity. Demanding a narrow and historically constructed understanding of identity not only misunderstands the political importance of diversities in sexuality, but relinquishes the particular strengths that obtain among same-sex practitioners who go under other names. This does not at all mean giving up the communities which have achieved strength and visibility as being positively gay; but to accept the idea that everyone else is duplicitously 'in the closet' is to hand over tremendous political power to the state. A heterosexist system has required us to name our partners and limit our sexuality to a narrow range of cross-gender behaviours. To demand a narrow gay identity, even implicitly, within safe-sex educational practices runs the risk of duplicating this form of oppression. To refuse to claim that everyone any of us has ever had sex with is, thereby, 'gay' is not to de-gay our community: rather, it is to complicate and confound heterosexuality, to create more space for sexual alliances, not less. Reclaiming sexual spaces and subcommunities in their own terms builds on the strength of queer culture without ceding the specific history and gains of urban gay communities – they are a vitally important form of queer culture, and in a unique position to channel resources to safe-sex projects, but they are not the only form.

It is strategically critical to continue asserting gay identity and gay community, but it is equally important to recognise that sexualities of resistance exist most importantly in their particularities of place and style, and not in adopting specific identities or relations to communities which identities imply. Safe-sex organising must work to open up sexual possibilities regardless of the names people choose for their pleasures.

NOTES

* This chapter was originally published in C. Patton (1996) *Fatal Advice*, Durham, NC: Duke University Press.

1 See, for example, the 'Facing AIDS' issue of *Radical America*, (Boston) 20:6, November/December 1987, which wonders 'whether the enormous amount of rage in the gay male community will ever find a political form' (p. 6), and an editorial in a subsequent issue devoted to AIDS (21:2–3, November/December 1988), which claimed that '1988 marked the beginning of a new national grass roots movement, an AIDS movement' (p. 3). By contrast, my *Sex and Germs: The Politics of AIDS* (Patton, 1985a), Dennis Altman's *AIDS in the Mind of America* (1986), a *New England Journal of Public Policy* special issue on AIDS (O'Malley, 1988), not to mention countless articles in lesbian and gay newspapers and magazines, clearly demonstrate that there was substantial activism concerning research, safe sex, discrimination, policy, ethics, and care as soon as the reports on the first cases were published in *Morbidity and Mortality Weekly Report*.

ACT UP is the now internationally-known acrynom for the AIDS Coalition to Unleash Power. Originally a New York City-based activist group principally concerned to criticize media and government inaction through highly visible direct action, the group soon saw 'chapters' in other American cities and around the world. As the sentiment spread, ACT UP groups diversified in their political tactics, drawing on both the sensational style of New York ACT UP, but also employing protest marches and sit-ins, as well as negotiating directly with government and, especially, drug company officials. Thus, ACT UP, and the various groups that split off from it (including Queer Nation and the Treatment Action Group, which focused on rereading data from clinical trials and cooperating in community research initiatives) is an evolving and variable form of social action.

2 For an analysis of the problems with temporal concepts in describing AIDS, see Erni (1994).

3 For discussion of right-wing responses see Patton (1985a, 1993), Altman (1986), and Watney (1987).
4 For a discussion of the emergence of lesbian and gay activism in the postwar era, see D'Emilio (1983).
5 AZT, or zidovudine, is the only fully approved anti-HIV drug.
6 In 1987, conservative US Senator Jesse Helms succeeding in passing an amendment to the law which distributed funding for AIDS research and education projects. This amendment prohibited money going to organisations that 'promote homosexuality or promiscuity'.
7 In the 1980s, young people in general seemed not to recognise themselves as the subjects of risk reduction advice. By the early 1990s some young gay men seemed to practise intercourse without condoms as a means of marking themselves as different from older gay men, or perhaps as dissidents from a national campaign of sexual austerity.

REFERENCES

Altman, Dennis (1986) *AIDS in the Mind of America*, New York: Doubleday.
Callen, Michael (ed.) (1988) *Surviving and Thriving with AIDS*, New York: PWA Coalition.
Callen, Michael and Berkowitz, Richard (1983) *How to Have Sex in an Epidemic*, New York: News From the Front Publications.
Centers for Disease Control (CDC) (1986) 'Classification system for human T-lymphotropic virus type III/lymphadenopathy-associated virus infections', *Morbidity and Mortality Weekly Report*, 35: 334–339.
D'Emilio, John (1983) *Sexual Politics, Sexual Community*, Chicago: University of Chicago Press.
Erni, John (1994) *Unstable Frontiers: Technomedicine and the Cultural Politics of 'Curing' AIDS*, Minneapolis: University of Minnesota Press.
Freire, Paolo (1973) *Education for Critical Consciousness*, New York: Seabury Press.
O'Malley, Padraig (ed.) (1988) *The AIDS Epidemic: Private Rights and the Public Interest*, Boston: Beacon Press.
Patton, Cindy (1985a) *Sex and Germs: The Politics of AIDS*, Boston: South End Press.
—— (1985b) 'Heterosexual AIDS panic: a queer paradigm', *Gay Community News*, 9 February.
—— (1993) '"Tremble heteroswine"', in Michael Warner (ed.) *Fear of a Queer Planet*, Minneapolis: University of Minnesota Press.
Redfield, R. *et al.*, (1986) 'The Walter Reed staging classification for HTLV-III/LAV infection', *New England Journal of Medicine*, 314: 131–132.
Watney, Simon (1987) *Policing Desire*, Minneapolis: University of Minnesota Press.

Chapter 9

The process of drug injection
Applying ethnography to the study of HIV risk among IDUs

Stephen Koester

In the introduction to *Making It Crazy*, an ethnography of discharged mentally ill patients, Sue Estroff explains participant observation, the methodological tradition of ethnography, as an attempt by an anthropologist 'to learn and reach understanding through asking, doing, watching, testing, and experiencing for herself the same activities, rituals, rules and meanings as the subjects. Our subjects become the experts, the instructors, and we become the students' (Estroff, 1981: 20). She concludes by cautioning that 'we are restricted in reaching optimal levels of experience and participation in the subjects' world if we are to remain sane' (1981: 20).

Those of us conducting ethnographic research among drug users are constrained from achieving Estroff's optimal level of participant observation for a variety of reasons, and while preserving our sanity may be one, others include legal, ethical and personal safety issues that accompany research on illicit drug use.

In spite of these constraints, a number of anthropologists and sociologists have applied the methodology and perspective of participant observation to the study of drug use and human immunodeficiency virus (HIV) transmission, and in so doing, have significantly enhanced our understanding of injection drug users' (IDU) lives and the behaviour that places many IDUs at increased risk of HIV infection. This chapter illustrates their contribution with a discussion of injection-related practices that may facilitate HIV transmission, but that unlike syringe sharing are often unrecognised and frequently misunderstood.[1]

Ethnography is particularly well-suited for understanding 'hidden' populations (Adler, 1985, 1990; Agar, 1986; Moore, 1993; NRC, 1989), and for designing public health strategies aimed at reducing the risk of disease among their members (Wiebel, 1988). As the term suggests, participant observation occurs in the natural setting; the ethnographer learns by being there, by seeing what people do, by listening to what they say and by experiencing at first hand the factors that influence their lives (Adler, 1993). The application of this methodological approach to the study of a behaviourally transmitted disease like AIDS provides the means for identifying behaviours that facilitate transmission, discovering the meaning of those behaviours to the people engaging in them, and understanding how contextual factors influence their occurrence.

Participant observation implies not only that the researcher engages in the everyday lives of people, but that the research is itself a participatory process. The comment by Estroff that the people we study are the experts and we are their students captures this notion. It suggests the dialogic character of fieldwork, the ongoing interaction of researcher and subject. This aspect of ethnographic research enables the researcher to gain an emic[2] or insider understanding of the phenomena being studied, and in applied research it enables the subject to inform intervention design.

In the late 1980s, a small number of researchers applying this research tradition began collecting evidence that while the sharing of a syringe between two or more IDUs may be the predominant injection-associated behaviour facilitating HIV transmission it may not be the only injection-associated practice that does so. Additional injection-associated risks may occur even when IDUs use separate syringes to inject. In the following, ethnography's contribution to our understanding of HIV transmission among IDUs is illustrated through a discussion of these findings. These additional injection-associated behaviours are identified, reasons for their occurrence are described and suggestions for interventions targeting these practices are discussed. These findings are the result of ongoing fieldwork among drug injectors in Denver, Colorado and a review of the literature. The Denver data was collected as part of two National Institute on Drug Abuse (NIDA) funded projects examining HIV interventions aimed at drug users. The author conducted research on this topic throughout the duration of these two projects, and in 1993 participated in the NIDA-funded multi-site Needle Hygiene project.[3] These ethnographic studies included ongoing interaction with IDUs in the natural settings in which they live, systematic observations of their injection practices and open-ended interviews about their lives, their drug use and the behaviours they engage in to acquire and use drugs.

THE PROCESS OF DRUG INJECTION

Several studies have reported injection-associated practices in addition to the direct transfer of a contaminated syringe that may contribute to the transmission of HIV among drug injectors (Grund *et al.*, 1989, 1990, 1991; Inciardi and Page, 1991; Jose *et al.*, 1993; Koester, 1989, 1993; Koester *et al.*, 1990; Needle *et al.*, 1994; Page, *et al.*, 1990; Samuels *et al.*, 1991; Zule, 1992). These practices occur as intermediate steps in the process of drug preparation and injection rather than at the point of injection, and they often occur as a consequence of the arrangements injectors make to obtain drugs (Koester and Hoffer, 1994). Behaviours included are the common use of injection-associated paraphernalia (water, cookers or drug mixing containers, and cotton filters) and the use of one syringe to mix, divide and distribute shared or jointly purchased drugs. In these practices the syringe is not shared; its contents are shared (Koester and Hoffer, 1994).

These behaviours appear to be regular, routinised components of the injection process. Because they occur as intermediate steps in this process, however, they are not as readily apparent or easy to conceptualise as the direct sharing of a syringe. Their potential role in HIV transmission remains unrecognised or only partially understood by many IDUs as well as by researchers examining injection-associated HIV risks. We have coined the term 'indirect sharing' to distinguish these possibly risky injection practices from the direct use of a single syringe by two or more IDUs and to suggest their more masked character (Koester and Hoffer, 1994).

Nine potentially contaminating 'indirect sharing' practices can be distinguished. These are: (1) rinsing previously used syringe(s) in a shared water container prior to drug preparation and injection; (2) using one participant's syringe to draw up water for dissolving the drug; (3) using the rubber, internal end of a participant's syringe plunger to mix water with the drug; (4) using one participant's syringe to measure and distribute drug solution shares to each participant; distribution then occurs through backloading, frontloading (methods of squirting the solution from the donor syringe into the receiving syringe), or by squirting the other users' shares back into the cooker; (5) drawing drug shares through a common cotton filter; (6) returning the drug solution to the common cooker or directly to another injector's syringe if an injector inadvertently draws up more than his/her share; (7) returning the drug solution to the cooker or directly into another's syringe to 'kick them out a taste'; (8) 'beating a cotton' that others have placed their needles in to draw up their dose; and (9) rinsing a used syringe in water in which others have previously placed used syringes for mixing and rinsing.

The nine injection-associated practices identified should not be considered as a complete inventory of potentially risky injection behaviours. As Bryan Page and his colleagues note, 'inter-community variations in self-injection practices are potentially infinite, and each variant may be accomplished by different kinds of risk of HIV infection' (Page et al., 1990). A variety of factors including the quality and quantity of the drug being injected, the way it was acquired, the social and physical setting in which it is used, and the ingenuity of the IDUs preparing it may affect the degree of HIV risk involved. Behaviours observed among IDUs in Denver, a Midwestern American city, may not encompass the range of injection-associated practices occurring elsewhere. For example, in Denver, frontloading – the squirting of the drug solution from one syringe into the hub connecting the needle and barrel of another syringe – does not occur because the most common syringes available do not have removable needles.

DRUG PREPARATION: MIXING, DIVIDING AND DISTRIBUTING

Potential HIV contamination may occur in a variety of ways and at various steps during the preparation of drugs. Water, cookers and cottons are sometimes shared even when each injector separately prepares their drug dose. This seems to occur most frequently with the water that injectors use for rinsing their syringes and dissolving the drug (Figure 9.1). Ethnographers in Denver observed situations in which a common container of water was used for rinsing syringes and/or mixing with the drug even though each injector was preparing their own individual dose in separate cookers. Frequently, however, water, as well as cottons and cookers, is shared when injectors divide and distribute a shared drug during the course of preparing it for injection.

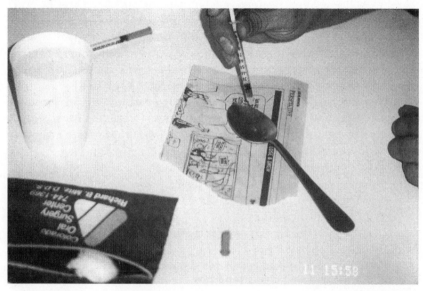

Figure 9.1 Basic drug injection paraphernalia: a disposable syringe, cotton for making a filter, a cup of water, and a drug mixing container or 'cooker'

Commonly injected drugs – heroin, cocaine or methamphetamine – can be divided and distributed in solid form prior to preparation for injection or after they have been dissolved into a liquid as part of the injection process. It is through this latter method of distribution that injectors are most likely to risk transmission of HIV or other blood-borne infections. Dividing and distributing the drug during the process of preparation and injection appears to occur most frequently when injectors buy small quantities of drugs for immediate use. This includes quantities of drugs that participants can consume at one time, either as single doses or in a sequence of doses taken over a short period of time. Examples include injectors who jointly purchase enough heroin to 'get well' or to get a 'fix', and injectors who buy a quantity of cocaine that they will consume together over the course of a single injection episode. Drugs are also transferred from one IDU's syringe to another IDU's syringe when one IDU gives another a 'taste', or small portion of their dose.

Step 1: Mixing

Typically, one injector takes responsibility for preparing and dividing the drug. This is often the person who contributed the most to the drug's purchase and/or the person who actually 'copped' or bought the drug from the 'connect' or dealer. This responsibility may also be delegated to the individual other injection participants feel is most proficient at drug preparation. The individual responsible for a shared drug's preparation places it in the cooker, and then, using their syringe (the donor syringe) draws up water and discharges it into the cooker (Figure 9.2). Generally, 10 to 25 units of water are drawn up for each injector. In some cases, IDUs measure the water using the calibrations on the donor syringe barrel, while at other times it is estimated. The drug is then stirred with the syringe plunger until it dissolves. When preparing heroin, the solution is sometimes heated by placing a match or cigarette lighter under the container for a few seconds.

HIV contamination is possible at this stage if: (1) the 'donor' syringe used

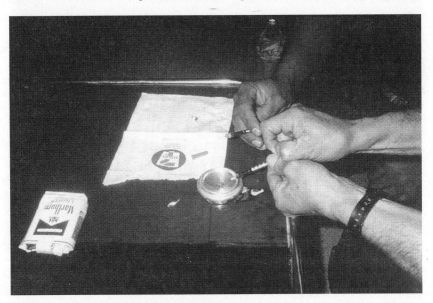

Figure 9.2 Using a common 'cooker' (drug mixing container) and drawing the shared drug solution through a common 'cotton' or filter

for drawing up the water has previously been used and not adequately disinfected. In this case, the contaminated bioburden – residue containing HIV infected blood – may be flushed out of the needle when the water for mixing is discharged into the cooker; or (2) the container of water used for mixing with the drug has previously been used for rinsing syringes or mixing drugs. In Denver, injectors frequently begin the injection process by rinsing their syringes once or twice with water. Usually this occurs before the water is used for mixing with the drug. The purpose of this pre-injection rinse is to lubricate the syringe and make sure it is working properly (Figure 9.3).

Step 2: Measuring and distributing shares

After the drug is mixed, a 'cotton' filter is placed in the cooker. Cigarette filters and cotton from a cotton swab are frequently used for this purpose. Using the syringe plunger, the individual preparing the drug pushes the cotton around the cooker to soak up the solution. The entire solution is then drawn through this filter and into the 'donor' syringe. The cotton 'captures' particles that might otherwise clog the syringe. Using the calibrations on the donor syringe barrel, this same injector measures the total amount of the drug to determine each injector's share. Once portions are calculated, the IDU preparing the drug distributes it by squirting all but their share of the solution back into the cooker or directly into the barrels of the other injectors' syringes. Some IDUs prefer this latter method, sometimes called backloading, because it saves time and eliminates the need to draw the drug through the cotton filter a second time, a step that may result in the loss of some of the drug (Figure 9.4). During this procedure HIV can be passed to other IDUs' syringes if the syringe used for measuring shares of the drug solution is contaminated with bioburden. The virus may be transferred if bioburden is flushed out of the needle when the drug solution is discharged into the mixing container or directly into other IDUs' syringes.

There are variations to the sequences described. For example, in some cases IDUs will measure the water for mixing the drug and not re-measure the drug solution. In these instances, the drug mixture is not drawn back into the donor syringe. Instead, it is left in the container for each injector to draw up his or her share (Figure 9.2). While this method reduces the number of times the liquid passes through the donor syringe, it does not necessarily decrease risk. Conceivably, HIV could be transferred by any needle touching the common filter and mixing container. In addition, when injectors draw their shares from a common container they frequently take more than their share. When this happens, the excess amount of the solution is discharged back into the container. This practice may result in the drug solution being contaminated, not only by the donor syringe, but by other injectors' syringes as well.

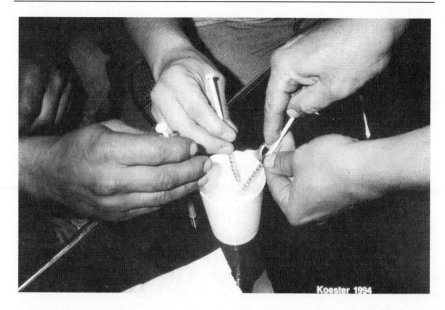

Figure 9.3 A common source of water used for (1) rinsing, lubricating and/or testing syringes prior to injection; (2) drawing up water to mix with the drug; (3) rinsing syringes immediately after injection

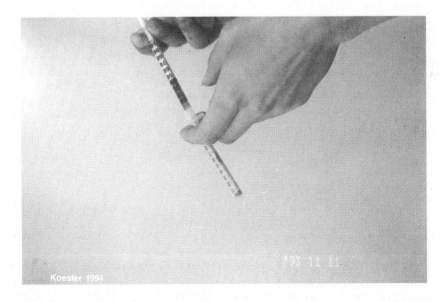

Figure 9.4 'Backloading', a method of transferring the drug solution from one syringe to another

ADDITIONAL RISKS: SHARING THROUGH COTTON FILTERS

Indirect sharing also occurs when an injector: (1) 'kicks a taste' back into the mixing container for another injector; (2) leaves a 'wet cotton' or a 'taste' in the mixing container for another injector; or (3) 'beats a cotton'. A 'taste' or 'wet cotton' is generally a small (less than half) portion of an individual's drug dose. This small amount is often exchanged for providing a service or extended to another injector who is unable to contribute to the purchase of the drug and/or is sick. Leaving another injector a taste or a wet cotton may promote HIV transfer because it is likely that the drug, or the water used to prepare it, has been in the syringe of the person supplying the drug, or that the drug has become contaminated from other IDUs placing their needles in the cotton and mixing container.

'Beating a cotton' is also a potential source of transmission. After the participating IDUs have withdrawn their shares from the cooker and injected, one of the them will attempt to squeeze any remaining drug solution from the cotton filter. This is accomplished by adding a small amount of water to the cooker, gently stirring it with the syringe plunger and then soaking it up with the cotton. The IDU then draws this solution into his or her syringe and injects. The drug solution that is drawn through the cotton may be a source of HIV because: (1) it may contain bioburden from the syringe used to mix and measure the solution; (2) other injectors' needles have come into contact with it; and (3) the water used to 'beat' it may have become contaminated because other injectors used the container for mixing their drug and rinsing their syringes. Some injectors do not 'beat cottons' because they do not believe there is sufficient drug left in the cotton to warrant it, and because they regard 'beating a cotton' as demeaning.

An individual's role or position within an injection group appears to be related to their degree of risk of HIV infection from syringe sharing and the indirect sharing practices described. Ethnographic findings suggest that certain norms or rules determine who prepares shared drugs for injection. This is significant because the person preparing the drugs is in a pivotal position regarding potential HIV transmission. Since this individual is most likely to use their own syringe to prepare the drugs it follows that they are at least risk of becoming infected during the drug preparation and injection process. At the same time, this individual is the greatest potential source of infection for those who subsequently inject the prepared drug solution.

WHY DO IDUs ENGAGE IN THESE PRACTICES?

These practices may occur with greater frequency than the sharing of syringes because: (1) drug injectors have a variety of reasons in addition to potential HIV contamination for not sharing syringes but few if any reasons not to engage in these practices; (2) these practices are efficient ways to prepare and divide shared drugs; (3) drug injectors may not perceive these procedures as contributing to HIV risk.

Most injectors would prefer to use new syringes. The needle on a disposable insulin syringe, the most common syringe used by injectors in the United States, becomes dull after only a few injections. This makes injections painful, and it makes it more difficult to 'hit' a vein. Used syringes are also susceptible to clogging, a predicament IDUs loathe (Carlson *et al.*, 1995; Koester, 1994). There are no equivalent self-interests which would discourage IDUs not to engage in indirect sharing behaviours. On the contrary, these practices appear to facilitate the efficient preparation of drugs so that they can be quickly injected. Unlike syringe sharing, these behaviours do not have any obvious drawbacks for those involved.

As was discovered with the direct transfer of used syringes among drug injectors, these injection-associated practices are frequently pragmatic responses to structurally imposed conditions. Syringes are re-used because they are scarce and they are scarce because states and municipalities enforce laws that prohibit them (Koester, 1994). Likewise, many injectors commonly risk HIV infection when preparing drugs because they buy drugs together, and they buy drugs together because they are poor.

To overcome the economic uncertainty that pervades their lives, IDUs employ extensive and opportunistic strategies based upon a variety of legal, quasi-legal and illegal activities, none of which are particularly secure or financially rewarding. As a result, injectors develop ways to obtain drugs even though they are short of cash. Among the most reliable ways to accomplish this are to: (1) form temporary partnerships, combine resources and jointly purchase a drug; (2) perform a service in exchange for a drug; and (3) rely on the kindness of others for a 'taste' of a drug. All three of these methods are regularly employed by drug injectors, and each one sets up conditions that lead to indirect sharing. Each method requires that the participants share the drugs they obtain. The indirect sharing procedures described are among the easiest and most efficient ways to accomplish this division. Dividing a drug as a solution permits injection episode participants to use the calibrations on the syringe for measuring shares, thus ensuring an equitable division. Dividing the drug as part of the injection process eliminates the extra step of first separating the drug into equivalent amounts, an important consideration for individuals who may be in withdrawal or whose privacy for engaging in this illegal activity may be only momentary.

IDUs mentioned a variety of other reasons why they prefer to mix all of a shared drug as a solution and then divide it. Some believed the overall effect is stronger when the entire quantity is mixed together. They also mentioned that preparing the entire quantity prior to division ensures that the compound the drug has been cut with is evenly distributed in the solution.

Dividing drugs during preparation may be more common among heroin injectors and IDUs who combine heroin and cocaine (speedball) than among cocaine injectors. To suppress withdrawal symptoms, heroin injectors waste little time between acquiring their drug and injecting it, and they must carefully calculate the dose necessary to 'get well'. Cocaine injectors reported that while they divide a shared drug during its preparation, they also divide small amounts of powder cocaine prior to liquefying it by 'eyeballing' equivalent shares.

REDUCING THE RISK OF INDIRECT SHARING

Few injectors seem cognisant of the potential risks these practices pose. IDUs who have participated in these ethnographic investigations in Denver were ethnically diverse, used different drugs, and were long-term injectors who self-reported rarely sharing syringes. In addition, the majority had been recruited into our HIV intervention programme prior to their interviews with the ethnographer. Their participation in this programme implies that they had received an intervention aimed at reducing HIV-associated risk behaviours. At a minimum, this consists of HIV testing, pre- and post-test counselling sessions which stress injection-related risks, access to bleach and condoms, and one or two detailed, structured questionnaires about their risk behaviour. Nonetheless, the drug injectors interviewed reported engaging in various indirect sharing practices. The following exchange illustrates their lack of awareness of these behaviours:

Ethnographer: 'Who shoots first?'
Informant: 'He'll draw it all up and shoot part of it back in the spoon. Then I'll draw up mine.'
Ethnographer: 'Now does he clean that syringe with bleach?'
Informant: 'No, but he's the only one that uses that particular rig [syringe].'

The ethnographic research summarised here suggests that indirect sharing may be a frequent, and perhaps integral, part of drug injection. In Denver, even long-term injectors were oblivious to the potential danger inherent in transferring shared drugs. Discussions with ethnographers in other cities, and more informal interviews with a large number of injectors throughout the Denver metropolitan area, support the conclusion that these indirect sharing behaviours are not an anomaly.

Current warnings about indirect sharing practices are often limited to prevention messages cautioning IDUs 'not to re-use or share cotton balls, cookers, rinse/wash water, and other drug preparation and injection equipment because they may be contaminated with blood' (CDC/CSAT/NIDA, 1993). Such prevention messages do not address the variety and complexity of behaviours in which these items are used. Instead, they focus on the drug paraphernalia rather than the process and context in which the sharing of these items occurs. Indirect sharing practices in which paraphernalia (water, cookers and cottons) are used in the process of sharing drugs need to be distinguished from situations in which these items, particularly water and cookers, are shared by injectors who separately prepare their own individual drug dose. This distinction is significant.

Recent virological research has detected HIV-1 DNA in syringes, cottons, cookers and water taken from shooting galleries in Miami, Florida (Shapshack *et al.* 1995). It would appear that when paraphernalia are used in common as a consequence of drug sharing the HIV risk may be equivalent to the direct sharing of needles. In these cases a potentially contaminated syringe's contents, including bioburden, are transferred from one syringe to another. This may be more dangerous than using a common container of water or a previously used mixing container.

Developing public health interventions that address the multiple ways these items can be 'shared' is an important challenge for HIV prevention. At a minimum, current messages advising IDUs not to share syringes, and to use bleach or other disinfectants in situations when syringes will be shared, must be extended to include detailed information on the potential risks of indirect sharing. Likewise, it is essential that bleach distribution programmes and needle exchange projects alert their clients about these additional risks, since they occur even though IDUs have their own syringes.

Detailed prevention messages should encourage IDUs not to share drugs or the paraphernalia they use for preparing and injecting drugs. If they do share or jointly purchase drugs, the drug should be divided and distributed in solid form prior to preparation for injection. IDUs should then prepare their own dose using their own syringe, a separate cooker, clean water that no one else has used and their own cotton. After they inject, the water should be thrown away, the cotton should be discarded and the cooker should be discarded or thoroughly cleaned.

IDUs' lives are rarely so organised or stable that they could consistently maintain these precautions. When these recommendations cannot be implemented other options are needed. These may include: (1) suggesting that IDUs keep a separate 'donor' syringe for preparing shared drugs. This syringe could be marked so that IDUs do not use it for injecting; (2) encouraging IDUs always to use a new, unused syringe for preparing shared drugs; and (3) when a new syringe is not available, making sure that the syringe used for preparing the drug has been disinfected. To ensure the effectiveness of this third option, IDUs should be encouraged to clean their syringes with bleach as a first step in drug preparation.

While these recommendations provide IDUs with guidelines for injecting more safely, they also suggest the need for interventions that address the context in which these injection-associated behaviours occur. Indirect sharing behaviours, are embedded within a complex social activity: the process of drug acquisition, preparation and injection. They occur as a result of the social arrangements IDUs construct to carry out these activities. Thus, interventions aimed at lessening them should go beyond the individual focus of many current intervention programmes and target the social groups within which these potentially risky practices take place.

The benefits of targeting social groups instead of individuals emerged during a focus group the author was conducting to determine IDUs' response to a revision of a syringe-hygiene protocol. The assembled IDUs were asked how they prepared their drugs, and specifically how they mixed, measured and distributed shared drugs. During the ensuing discussion, an injector suddenly said, 'Oh shit, I think I see what you're getting at. Man, we're still sharing even though we're using our own fits [syringes].' This injector's sudden insight was quickly picked up by other focus group participants. They too understood the implications, and with alacrity began talking about other possible drug preparation and injection-associated risks. This experience indicated that injectors may not realise how infections are transmitted and that intervention messages telling them what not to do are insufficient. It also suggested that working with injectors in a participatory, problem-solving format could be an effective intervention. It may be efficient and cost effective as well, since several injectors can be intervened with at a time and the information rapidly disseminated. This interactive approach may be most effective with injection networks; groups of people who regularly cooperate in the process of obtaining, sharing and injecting drugs. Their familiarity with each other may encourage more open discussion and provide a structure for implementing and reinforcing risk reduction.

By focusing on these social groups or drug injection networks, we can demonstrate to their members that they have a mutual self-interest in learning about the behaviours that place them at risk and in devising strategies to avoid them. An assumption behind this approach is that members of injection networks will change, not only because of the social support they provide each other, but also out of mutual self-interest. Discussing injection-associated risk behaviours with IDUs who engage in these activities together may help promote the idea that the behaviour of one can affect (and possibly infect) others. This model seems particularly important for the indirect sharing practices described here because they occur in numerous and complex arrangements, and because they are not always obvious to those engaging in them.

This proposed injection network intervention builds upon current interventions like the 'Indigenous Leader' model developed by Wayne Wiebel, and, like that model, it developed during the course of ethnographic research (Wiebel, 1988). In the Indigenous Leader model, IDUs are encouraged by community-health outreach workers to discuss the behaviours that may place them at risk of HIV and to identify ways in which they can lessen those risks (see Chapter 12). In this proposed network intervention the 'individual risk assessment' is extended to include the social group in which these risks occur. The assumption behind this adaptation is that socially embedded risk behaviours require socially based interventions. In this model the emphasis of intervention shifts from individual to group risk reduction. Trained interventionists employing a focus group format encourage members of injection networks to realise their interdependence and to develop ways of modifying the behaviours that place them at risk. Indigenous outreach workers augment these group discussions and reinforce attempts at risk reduction through ongoing contact with network members.

Conceptually, this participatory, socially oriented intervention model borrows from the perspective and methods of ethnography. It applies the 'subject as teacher' notion described by Estroff, toward understanding HIV risk behaviour and developing strategies to lessen it, and it incorporates the dialogic, participatory elements of ethnographic methods to construct a public health intervention. It assumes that important insights will emerge from open discussions among intervention participants, and between part-icipants and trained facilitators. From these discussions, members of injection networks can reach greater understanding of the behaviours that place them at risk of HIV infection, and together they can develop ways to lessen those risks. This social model also incorporates ethnography's emphasis on context by extending risk reduction to include the circumstances that influence risky behaviour. It assumes that a group of behaviourally linked individuals will have greater success in altering the conditions and situations that lead to risk than will individual IDUs. Together, injectors can develop methods for overcoming the multiple contextual hurdles that impede harm reduction.

CONCLUSION

Ever since the link between injection drug use and HIV was recognised over a decade ago, the overwhelming emphasis of behavioural research and public health prevention efforts aimed at IDUs has been on syringe sharing, the direct transfer of a single syringe between two or more IDUs. In contrast, the possible yet subtler avenues for infection described here have remained obscure, and in many cases unrecognised. With the inclusion of ethnographic research as an integral component of HIV epidemiology, our understanding of both syringe sharing and these other potential injection-associated risks has increased significantly. Ethnographic research on the context in which IDUs share syringes has refuted the notion that needle sharing is best understood as either a bad personal habit or an exotic subcultural ritual (Koester, 1994), and, as described here, ethnographic research on the process of drug injection has revealed a range of injection-associated practices that may place IDUs at risk of HIV even when they use their own syringes to inject.

Perhaps the most alarming of these lesser-known injection risks occurs when IDUs share drugs, and specifically, when they divide a shared drug as a solution during preparation for injection. This practice appears to be common among injectors observed and interviewed in Denver. It may lead to HIV transmission if the syringe used for preparing and dividing the shared drug is contaminated with HIV. Transmission may occur because, during distribution, bioburden, including HIV, is transferred with the drug solution from the contaminated syringe to a common drug-mixing container or directly into other IDUs' syringes. It appears unlikely that this intermediate injection step in which the contaminated drug solution is first transferred to another syringe or momentarily placed in a mixing container and then drawn into other IDUs' syringes significantly reduces the risk of HIV transmission.

To counter these injection-associated risks requires an intervention approach that is based on a thorough understanding of how and why these risks take place. The realisation that these risky behaviours often occur as a consequence of the social arrangements IDUs construct to acquire drugs suggests the need for interventions that are also social, both in concept and implementation. The model proposed here is an example of such an approach. It promotes behaviour change at the level of the injection network rather than the individual, and it does so by bringing members of a network together and encouraging them to actively participate in identifying and overcoming the behaviours and circumstances that place them at risk.

The relatively recent identification of the injection associated HIV risks discussed in this chapter suggests the benefit of making participant observation, the in-depth study of human behaviour in the natural setting, an integral part of epidemiological research. As Bryan Page and his colleagues have advised:

> Intervention to prevent the subtler gateways of contagion needs to be based on detailed understanding of the behaviours it seeks to change and through cultural understanding of the contexts in which these behaviours occur.
>
> (Page *et al.*, 1990: 69)

This chapter has attempted to demonstrate the critical role ethnographic research has played in accomplishing these tasks. The potentially risky practices reported and the tentative guidelines outlined for lessening their potential HIV risk emerged from the participatory nature of the ethnographic method, the interplay of observation and open-ended interviews, and of the researcher and the subject. This integral aspect of ethnographic research not only provided a window into the lives of others, it also allowed those others the opportunity to inform the research. The explanations and insights regarding the behaviours described emerged from ongoing discussions with IDUs. Their 'indigenous' knowledge provided an understanding of why these practices occur, as well as suggestions for addressing them.

NOTES

1 This chapter incorporates aspects of two previous articles by the author. See Koester (1995) and Koester and Hoffer (1994).

2 Some anthropologists use the term emic to describe their effort to understand a culture or group from the perspective of its members.

3 The first of these NIDA-funded studies (1988–90) was a subcontract with the University of Illinois-Chicago. Dr Wayne Wiebel was the principal investigator. This was a demonstration of the Indigenous Leader model for HIV intervention (Wiebel, 1988). The second NIDA study (1991–95) was a cooperative agreement (DA–06912). It compared two HIV intervention models. The principal investigator of this study was Robert Booth, PhD. NIDA has frequently supported ethnographic research on drug use and has been instrumental in advocating multi-site ethnographic studies. The Needle Hygiene Study (NIDA contract no. 271–90–8400, July 1993) is one of the most recent. Several anthropologists and sociologists were involved in this study. In addition to the author working in Denver, they included: Michael Clatts, PhD (New York), Laurie Price, PhD (Flagstaff, Arizona), Ann Finlinson, PhD (San Juan, Puerto Rico), Ricky Bluthenthal (Oakland, CA), and Todd Pierce (Hartford, CT). The study was coordinated by Carol Anglin. The Community Research Branch of the National Institute on Drug Abuse, under the direction of Richard Needle, PhD, sponsored the project, and Helen Cesari was the project officer.

REFERENCES

Adler, P. (1985) *Wheeling and Dealing: An Ethnography of an Upper-Level Drug Dealing and Smuggling Community*, New York: Columbia University Press.

Adler, P. (1990) 'Ethnographic research on hidden populations: Penetrating the drug world', in *The Collection and Interpretation of Data from Hidden Populations*, National Institute on Drug Abuse Research Monograph 98, Washington, DC: Department of Health and Human Services Publication No.(98) 96–112.

Adler, P. (1993) 'Ethnography and epidemiology: Building bridges', in *Epidemiologic Trends in Drug Abuse: Proceedings of the Community Epidemiology Working Group* June 1993, US Government Printing Office 531–543: NIH No. 93–3645.

Agar, M. (1986) *Speaking of Ethnography*. Beverly Hills, CA: Sage Publications.

Agar, M. (1993) 'Ethnography: an aerial view', in *Epidemiologic Trends in Drug Abuse: Proceedings of the Community Epidemiology*, Working Group June 1993, US Government Printing Office 520–530: NIH No. 93–3645.

Carlson, R. G., Siegal, H.A. and Falck, R.S. (1995) 'Ethnography, epidemiology and public policy: Needle use practices and risk reduction among IV drug users in the midwest', in D.A. Feldman (ed.) *Anthropology and Global AIDS Policy*, Westport, CT: Greenwood Press.

CDC/CSAT/NIDA (Centers for Disease Control, Center for Substance Abuse Treatment and the National Institute on Drug Abuse) (1993) *HIV/AIDS Prevention Bulletin*, April 19. US Department of Health and Human Services, Washington, DC.

Estroff, S. (1981) *Making It Crazy*, Berkeley: University of California Press.

Grund, J.P.C., Kaplan, C. and Adriaans, N. (1989) 'Needle exchange and drug sharing: A view from Rotterdam', *Newsletter of the International Working Group on AIDS and IV Drug Use*, 4(1): 4–5.

Grund, J.P.C., Kaplan, C., Adriaans, N. *et al.* (1990) 'The limitations of the concept of needle sharing: The practice of frontloading', *AIDS*, 4: 819–821.

Grund, J.P.C., Kaplan, C., Adriaans, N. and Blanken, P. (1991) 'Drug sharing and HIV transmission risks: The practice of frontloading in the Dutch injecting drug user population', *Journal of Psychoactive Drugs*, 23(1): 1–10.

Inciardi, J. A. and Page, J.B. (1991) 'Drug sharing among intravenous drug users', *AIDS*, 5(6): 772–773.

Jose, B., Friedman, S. R., Neaigus, A. (1993) 'Syringe-mediated drug-sharing (backloading): A new risk factor among injecting drug users', *AIDS*, 7: 1653–1660.

Koester, S. (1989) 'Water, cookers and cottons: Additional risks for intravenous drug abusers', in *Epidemiologic Trends in Drug Abuse: Proceedings of the Community Epidemiology Working Group*, June 1989, US Government Printing Office, 00768: 118–120.

Koester, S. (1993) 'Ethnography and high risk drug use', in *Problems of Drug Dependence, 1992: Proceedings of the 54th Annual Scientific Meeting*, National Institute on Drug Abuse Monograph 132, Washington, DC: Department of Health and Human Services Publication No. 93–3505–132.

Koester, S. (1994) 'Copping, running and paraphernalia laws: Contextual variables and needle risk behaviour among injection drug users in Denver', *Human Organization*, 53(3): 287–295.

Koester, S. (1995) 'Applying the methodology of participant observation to the study of injection related risks', in R. Ashery and E. Lambert, *Qualitivate Methods in Drug Abuse and HIV Research*, National Institute on Drug Abuse Research Monograph, Washington, DC: National Institute of Health.

Koester, S. and Hoffer, L. (1994) 'Indirect sharing: Additional HIV risks associated with drug injection', *AIDS and Public Policy Journal*, 9(2): 100–105.

Koester, S., Booth, R. and Wiebel, W. (1990) 'The risk of HIV transmission from sharing water, drug-mixing containers and cotton filters among intravenous drug users', *InternationalJournal of Drug Policy*, 1(6): 28–30.

Moore, D. (1993) 'Ethnography and illicit drug use: Dispatches from an anthropologist in the field', *Addiction Research*, 1: 11–25.

National Research Council (NRC) (1989) *AIDS: Sexual Behaviour and Intravenous Drug Use*, C. F. Turner, H. G. Miller, and L. E. Moses (eds). Washington, DC: National Academy Press, 186–240.

Needle, R., Cesari, H., Koester, S., Clatts, M., Price, L., Bluthenthal, R., Finlinson, A., and Pierce, T. (1994) 'Multi-person use of drug injection equipment: HIV transmission risks associated with drug preparation and injection practices', paper presented at Tenth International Conference on AIDS, Yokohama, Japan.

Page, J. B., Chitwood, D., Smith, P., Kane, N., and McBride. D. (1990) 'Intravenous drug use and HIV infection in Miami', *Medical Anthropology Quarterly*, 4(4): 56–71.

Samuels, J. F., Vlahov, D., Anthony, J.C. (1991) "The practice of 'frontloading" among intravenous drug users: Association with HIV-antibody', *AIDS*, 5: 343.

Shapshak, P., McCoy C. B., Shah, S. M., Rivers, J. E., Weatherby, N. L, Chitwood D. D. *et al*. (1995) 'The detection of HIV-1 in needle/syringes, paraphernation and washes from shooting galleries in Miami: combating the risk for HIV infection in IDU women', paper presented at the HIV Infection in Women Conference, Washington DC, February 22–24.

Wiebel, W. (1988) 'Combining ethnographic and epidemiologic methods in targeted AIDS interventions: The Chicago model', in R. Battjes and R. Pickens (eds) *Needle Sharing among Intravenous Drug Abusers: National and International Perspectives*, National Institute on Drug Abuse Research Monograph 80, Washington, DC: Department of Health and Human Services Publication 137–150.

Zule, W. A. (1992) 'Risk and reciprocity: HIV and the injection drug user', *Journal of Psychoactive Drugs*, 24(3): 243–249.

Chapter 10

Promoting risk management among drug injectors

Robert Power

This chapter sets out to explore four interrelated assertions concerning injecting drug use and the risk of infectious disease. First, that there is a need for community-based interventions to effect behaviour change amongst injecting drug users. Second, that a prerequisite for any such interventions is an understanding of the lifestyles and daily routines of the target populations. Third, that some form of risk management, especially that related to injecting behaviour, is an integral component of many drug user lifestyles. Fourth, that we should seek to build on positive activities that are already part of daily routines and seek to discourage those that are prejudicial to risk reduction.

These assertions need to be placed in context. They derive from research conducted into the English drug scene of the mid-1990s. This is a time where needle and syringe schemes have been widely available for nearly a decade and have been proven to be largely effective in reducing the spread of HIV disease amongst injecting drug users (Dolan *et al.*, 1993). It is a time when outreach work is being challenged for being too closely focused on the individual drug user, for promoting individual change and for failing to penetrate networks of drug injectors far removed from treatment contact (ACMD, 1993). It is an era where risk management and harm minimisation are the prevailing paradigms and where community change is promoted as the desired outcome.

It is the matter of risk and risk management that is central to the concerns of this chapter. Not that any one of us is immune to risk. Modern life is a risky business and we all employ either personal or corporate risk management strategies as part of our daily routines. In his recent book on the subject, Adams (1995) points out that in the rapidly changing contemporary world, many of the old political, institutional and economic certainties have been undermined. Consequently, nothing much can be taken for granted and the notion of risk management is becoming a part of many facets and levels of modern life. He goes on to suggest that the context of risk management in the very-late-twentieth century is characterised by knowledge rather than ignorance. This contention stands up well to what we know about the poor match between knowledge of the risk of HIV transmission and sexual and drug injecting behaviour. A similar generalisable point had already been made by Beck (1993), who noted that our technological advances have meant that risk is not so much a consequence of natural and external forces, but more a result of social exigencies. To pursue the AIDS illustration, it is not that we do not possess the technology to combat HIV infection (sterile injecting equipment and condoms), but rather that social conditions and interactions mediate between their availability and effective use.

It is these social behavioural factors that we need to investigate in order to promote effective risk management. The health-related risks facing a drug injector, and the social and contextual variables involved, differ from those of people who pursue other lifestyles or pastimes. Hence, the risks and risk management variables relevant to injecting drug users are different in essence from those confronting mountaineers or mercenaries.

As pointed out by a number of commentators, there is a wide range of circumstantial, situational and social factors that will influence individual and group attitudes and responses towards risks related to drug injecting (Power, et al., 1988; McKeganey and Barnard, 1992; Grund et al., 1992). Although individual choice concerning risk and health behaviour is important, this cannot be dissociated from peer groups, social etiquette and social and community norms (Friedman et al., 1990; Booth and Wiebel, 1992; Burt and Stimson, 1993; Rhodes, 1993). Furthermore, Ouellet et al. (1991), through ethnographic observations in shooting galleries in Chicago, provide an example of the importance of situational and organisational factors in determining the risks associated with injecting.

The direct corollary of all this is that, to be most effective, interventions aimed at producing desired behaviour change must look beyond the individual. Just as risk management strategies are seated in the context of more or less complex social relations, so interventions need to be cognisant of the structure and activities of the resultant 'communities' or groups, however loosely defined these may be.

At one level, a 'community' can be seen to exist according to shared interests and activities and can be centred either on a specific geographic location or on social networks. Our research observations suggest that a common factor binding any social network or group of illicit drug users is the need to procure and consume an illicit product. Hence much of the communal activity of drug users, be it spatial or social, is primarily focused on the purchasing and consumption processes within the drug market.

RESEARCH CAN INFORM INTERVENTIONS

In relation to developing effective community-based services for drug injectors, the researcher and interventionist have interlinked roles. The task of the researcher is to describe and interpret the social meanings that underpin drug user behaviour (especially, in our context in relation to risk management, or mismanagement). It is for the interventionist to use these data (which may be both epidemiological and ethnographic) to develop interventions that are truly relevant to the groups they are targeting. This not only means interventions that are geared to the profiles of the recipients. They should also utilise the informal risk management structures and strategies that exist within the populations and ensure that interventions dovetail with their lifestyles and daily routines.

The data that inform the discussion in this chapter derive from a two-year study (funded by the UK Department of Health) of one hundred regular polydrug users, the majority of whom reported heroin as their drug of choice (Power, 1995). Respondents, who were not in direct contact with treatment agencies or other drug services provision, were recruited by snowballing through key contacts at three sites in England. Lifestyle, drug use and behavioural data were collected through a mix of research techniques that included semi-structured interviews, focus groups, and participant observation. One of the study aims was to investigate the types of coping strategies that were used in the daily lives of drug injectors to reduce the risk of infectious disease. It soon became apparent that individual choice, be it around drug purchasing and consumption or risk management, was seldom conducted in isolation, but was influenced and mediated by a number of contextual variables including peer pressure and peer norms and the setting and location of activity.

I want to use these data to stress the importance of drug users' social networks and their settings for developing community-based interventions. The data show the potential for interventions to operate on a number of levels. At one level interventions can build on the social structures and relationships that already exist amongst drug injectors. At another, they can integrate and encourage the positive aspects of risk management or protective strategies identified amongst networks. At a third level they can identify, target and discourage negative or high-risk behaviours. At yet another level they can focus on the infrastructure of the drug market itself as a vehicle for intervention and as a means of effecting desired change. I will conclude by suggesting that the shape and constituency of the intervention should be largely dependent upon its ultimate aims and objectives, as well as upon the populations or arenas that are to be targeted.

INTERVENTIONS SHOULD BUILD ON THE STRUCTURES OF DRUG USER SOCIAL NETWORKS

The key single variable that binds drug user relationships is the functional necessity to maintain drug supplies. The study showed this to be particularly the case amongst heroin users, where the daily need to procure drugs led to networks that were more cohesive and interdependent than those of stimulant-using groups, where intermittent bingeing was more common. The relative cohesiveness of these networks was found to be influenced by factors such as drug type, local drug economies, population density and wider drug trends. Furthermore, it was noted that the existence of street drug scenes in the large cities contrasted with smaller towns and rural areas. At the level of drug types, it was observed that much of the heroin dealing took place in private homes, whereas amphetamine sulphate distribution outlets tended to be centred more on semi-public venues such as public houses.

Opiate injectors tended to describe reciprocal and supportive relationships, that were often fluid, leading to overlap between differing networks of users. Functional reciprocity that was based on current purchasing and consumption patterns was seen to be threatened in times of shortage of supplies, when users were forced to act more individualistically. Yet, even in these circumstances, drug users relied on others, if not for actual drug supplies, then for relevant information.

As with any 'community' or network of social groups, some form of information dissemination is crucial to its functioning and existence. In this respect illicit drug users are no exception. Many referred to informal, word of mouth, information networks or 'grapevines', that acted as important media for communicating information on drug availability, quality and prices, and often linked differing networks. These grapevines were particularly important in times of supply shortages, when drug users would seek out others for much-needed information. From the perspective of the public health agenda, the same conduits can be utilised to disseminate health promotion materials.

Our data also revealed the importance of certain rules that bound networks and operated to regulate their successful functioning. Amongst some networks, certain behaviours (like being too chaotic) were considered grounds for exclusion from the group and its support mechanisms. One network in London exemplified this point. This group was well-established and was founded on the sale and consumption of heroin and cocaine. The core membership (including the dealer) was made up of established users, who would pass on advice and information to the new and casual recruits to the network. Such wisdom would include warnings about the dangers of needle use and sharing, inappropriate drug combinations and the mechanisms of seeking help. All this would be delivered spasmodically, informally and in the general context of getting on with the main business of buying, selling and consuming drugs. Even though persistently chaotic members were eventually excluded from the network, there were health gains for these individuals. A positive aspect of this rule of exclusion was that informal health education had the potential to be diffused to other groups of drug users, who were more chaotic in their lifestyles and often younger both in years and drug careers.

By identifying and describing key features in the structure and operation of drug user networks or 'communities' we can inform the development of targeted initiatives, especially those relying upon models of peer intervention. In terms of community-based interventions we need also to examine the potential to develop existing roles within networks, especially where these function to promote risk management. For example, in the network described above the drug dealer actively discouraged injecting amongst her customers. The dealer herself had experienced health problems as a result of injecting and now only smoked drugs. On several occasions she (along with her assistant and other core members of the group) was observed to remonstrate with others in the network over the dangers of injecting. Such key opinion leaders, especially those already engaged in informal peer education, should be utilised to full potential in community-based interventions.

This network by no means represents a unique scenario in terms of informal health advocacy. One heroin dealing couple recounted how, over time, they had passed on information concerning a treatment centre (that the husband had attended) to upwards of thirty in their network. The husband taught new injectors the best techniques of injecting, and felt that people listened to him because he was well-respected amongst drug user circles in the town. More generally, it was common for drug dealers to provide clean needles and syringes to their customers.

INTERVENTIONS SHOULD ENCOURAGE POSITIVE ASPECTS OF INFORMAL RISK MANAGEMENT

By examining the lifestyles of illicit drug users it soon became apparent that control strategies and risk management were a part of their daily routines. Health issues aside, the data highlighted the ways in which drug injectors adopted strategies to manage the risk of being without a supply of drugs.

It was common for drug users to purchase drugs in small quantities. They also reported dividing up drugs into smaller portions and rationing supply. Prescribed drugs (such as methadone and Dexedrine) were commonly obtained to be shared, bartered or sold in times of shortage or as alternatives to the primary drug. Additionally, many drug users reported adopting informal coping strategies to control their drug use patterns. For instance, regular heroin users commonly reported taking periodic breaks from drug use by leaving the area where they lived. Such strategies were not adopted in isolation, as leaving the area often involved staying with non-drug-using friends or family. These points indicate that risk management is by no means anathema to drug users and forms an integral part of their daily lives. Hence, it is not surprising that coping and risk management strategies were seen to be part of daily routines in relation to injecting practices.

Although none of our respondents were syringe exchange clients, ensuring a supply of new equipment and re-using syringes were the most popular strategies employed to reduce the likelihood of sharing. The main source of new injecting equipment was from a pharmacy, followed by a dealer (who may well have been a friend). Amongst injectors who commonly re-used their injecting equipment, personalising their equipment to prevent accidental sharing was a popular strategy (see also Burt and Stimson, 1993).

Other strategies adopted to reduce the likelihood of syringe sharing included: storing spare needles and syringes around the house; leaving injecting equipment with non-using friends; and making efforts to replenish supplies when down to the last needle and syringe in a pack.

Taking measures to clean injecting equipment was common, though rarely efficient. The most popular method was flushing or rinsing with water, which was most often done when re-using one's own syringe. Some injectors adopted a more rigorous cleaning method if they were to use another's syringe. Bleach or disinfectant was used only by a small minority to clean their equipment, mainly those who used their drugs in the privacy of their own homes. The majority placed greater emphasis on the provision of sterile equipment, rather than the process of disinfection.

One clear role for any form of community-based intervention would be to encourage, promote and build on those positive health behaviours and risk management strategies that already form part of the lifestyles and daily routines of drug users.

INTERVENTIONS SHOULD DISCOURAGE BEHAVIOURS THAT ARE PREJUDICIAL TO RISK MANAGEMENT

On the other hand, community-based interventions need to recognise and devise strategies to discourage and alter behaviours that are prejudicial to risk reduction. Some of these behaviours will be directly related to the availability of needles and syringes, others to the social contexts in which injecting takes place and the social meanings attached to such episodes. In each of these scenarios, community-based interventions need to be targeted towards discouraging high-risk activity and promoting appropriate risk management strategies.

Our data showed that the lack of availability of sterile injecting equipment was linked with several factors that commonly led to needle and syringe sharing. These factors, which echo observations that have been noted since the mid-1980s, included: being in a sexual relationship with another drug injector; the immediate need to use drugs (especially at night); withdrawal symptoms; intoxication; and being in situations (such as prison) or in areas (such as unfamiliar drug dealing arenas) where injecting equipment was scarce. Concerning this last point, isolation or exclusion from social networks was liable to lead to high-risk activity, such as purchasing and consuming drugs at street scenes.

Whereas it was common for drug users to adopt risk management strategies around the use of needles and syringes, the majority of the injectors in the study reported the sharing of injecting paraphernalia, such as filters and spoons. Both spoons and filters (which were often cigarette filters or cotton buds) were used in the preparation and consumption of injectable drugs. In order to block particulate matter, the drug passes through a 'filter' and into the needle and syringe. These filters are valued for the residue of drug that remains after this process has been completed. Sharing spoons and filters was commonly viewed as representing little risk. This practice was compounded by reports that drug users were wary of carrying injecting paraphernalia on their person, as it was felt that this could be used as evidence against them if they were arrested. Filters were saved as an emergency drug supply in times of shortage and evidence was found of filters being used as a currency for the purchase of other drugs, particularly pharmaceutical ones.

Furthermore, the sharing of injecting paraphernalia was a direct consequence of the common practice of drug users pooling resources to purchase drugs. Once drugs were obtained they were most often prepared and distributed communally, a process that not only included front- or back loading, but also entailed sharing filters and spoons.

Aside from these pragmatic reasons for sharing paraphernalia, social etiquette and community norms played an important part in the sharing of filters. Drug users would often find themselves injecting in another drug user's house. Amongst some networks of injectors it was common practice, after an injecting occasion, to leave used filters behind for the host. This was both a courtesy and payment in kind.

These examples highlight the need for change to be concentrated at the level of social relations and to focus on the norms that bind networks: in other words, interventions that are not primarily centred on the individual and individual change.

DRUG ARENAS PRESENT OPPORTUNITIES FOR COMMUNITY-BASED INTERVENTIONS

The city has often been the site for the study of illicit drug use and drug markets (see Johnson *et al.*, 1985; Parker *et al.*, 1987; Bean and Wilkinson, 1988). This section will indicate the way in which the drug markets that evolve and develop within urban areas offer particular opportunities for community-based interventions.

One of the main distinguishing features of city life is anonymity. In contrast with less urban areas, the city (and especially the metropolis and large conurbations) contains a population density that affords a degree of anonymity and urban spread that results in a plethora of public, semi-public and private drug markets that can be absorbed into its everyday life.

For instance, London has well-established drug scenes, well-known to regular users of illicit drugs. These venues can range from a particular neighbourhood or set of streets to public or semi-public venues, such as railway stations or pubs and clubs. Other drug dealing sites will be constantly shifting private addresses and other private and exclusive venues known only to drug users. Once identified and described, these venues can be incorporated into community-based interventions. By way of illustration, I will focus mainly on some recent research studies conducted in the London area.

Major metropolitan train stations have always created the conditions to foster popular drug markets. One such site in London was 'Trainstop'. Although under constant police surveillance, the wide range of seemingly ceaseless activity made it possible for illicit drug dealing to occur largely unseen. Amidst the bustle of commuting and constant interactions, arrivals and departures, numerous drug deals take place, on the concourse or in other public areas.

Whereas the most obvious signs of drug purchasing and consumption resulted in local protest and police activity, much of the everyday activity of the drug market would proceed unnoticed. The fast-food outlet adjacent to the station was also a place where drugs were dealt and where prostitutes (many of whom were drug injectors) met. In its toilets, drug users were observed to inject (often using the water from the toilet bowl to prepare their drugs for injection), and to clean their needles and syringes. The grocer's shop on the opposite corner was observed to be selling sterile needles and syringes to the drug users.

An interventionist, armed with these research observations, can view this picture from a different perspective and take advantage of the structures and locations that make up this particular drug market. To begin with, outreach workers can develop relationships with the key players. The outreach worker can spend regular sessions at the fast-food bar getting to know and gaining the trust of the drug using clientele. They might enlist and encourage the street-level drug dealers to pass on health information to their customers. They could ask the grocer to hand out leaflets on safe injecting with each syringe that he sells. They might even suggest working closely and non-judgmentally with him to ensure that the drug users get night and day access to the equipment they require. In other words, the researcher and outreach worker cooperate closely to superimpose the interventionist world on the world of the drug market, which is itself already grafted on to the world of the railway station.

This kind of community outreach approach, which was strongly promoted in the USA in the absence of freely available needles and syringes, has much potential in fine-tuning community change aimed at drug injectors (Wiebel, 1988; Ouellet et al., 1991; Murphy and Waldorf, 1991; Friedman, 1993). Once the confidence, trust and cooperation of such key role players have been gained, then health education and prevention materials can be routinely supplied and promoted at appropriate venues, and outreach workers can operate openly in engaging drug users. This potential is increased at venues such as Trainstop, where drug users would commute to the station from outlying areas in order to procure drugs and then return home. Such mobility and movement between overlapping drug user networks creates unique opportunities for the diffusion of peer education.

ROLES WITHIN THE DRUG MARKET CAN ASSIST COMMUNITY INTERVENTIONS

The roles occupied by drug users in the drug market itself open up opportunities for health advocacy and risk management promotion that can spread amongst differing networks. The drug markets in large cities employ and engage a wide range of individuals. These roles are often casual, and there is a high turnover. Most notable is the role of the small-scale user–dealer, a position held to a lesser or greater degree by most regular drug users at various times during their drug careers. Such user–dealers also operate as 'runners' (or assistants to those dealing in larger quantities of drugs). These 'runners' are the retailers or street vendors who have direct contact with the customers.

A similar structure was described in a recent study that focused on the distribution and purchasing of cocaine and crack in Britain (Green et al., 1994; Power et al., 1995). As well as street-based 'runners', ethnographic work identified others who acted as bicycle couriers providing a mobile service in illicit drugs.

As well as drug dealers who already operate as informal health advocates, we need to look at ways in which those involved in the drug market and who have wide access to other drug users can be integrated into community-based interventions. Outreach workers are well-placed to identify knowledgeable and respected individuals who can be approached and recruited as 'indigenous advocates' (Power, 1994).

CONCLUSION

At any given time there will always be a substantial proportion of illicit drug users not in contact with established services. Consequently, we need to develop community-based outreach that is relevant to their needs and which offers services that fit into their lifestyles and daily routines. The data outlined above show that many drug users' lives are characterised by communal activities and engagement with others. These activities may be largely functional and pragmatic, but they nevertheless bind their participants into loosely knit and often overlapping communities or social networks. Although ultimately risk management operates at the level of the individual, nodal points can be identified (both in terms of activities and locations) where communal behaviour either enhances or detracts from effective risk management or control strategies. So, for example, the sharing of injecting paraphernalia was influenced both by the exigencies of the drug market and by the social etiquette and cultural norms that underpinned injecting practices. Similarly, it was noted that the proclivity to share injecting equipment was influenced by a diversity of factors that ranged from states of intoxication to relationship with sexual partner, and situational variables, such as imprisonment.

By describing and examining the structure and everyday activities and lifestyles of these drug using networks we can point to precise behaviours that need to be encouraged, discouraged or altered. For instance, ensuring a regular informal supply of sterile injecting equipment (from whatever source), and the strategies already adopted by social networks to facilitate this, should be encouraged. On the other hand, the practice of sharing injecting paraphernalia, such as filters and spoons, which has become part of the social etiquette of certain groups of drug injectors, needs to be actively discouraged. As outlined above, there are other behaviours that need modifying or altering, such as ineffective sterilisation of injecting equipment.

Now the question that is begged is: how do we best achieve these particular objectives? There has been much debate in recent years around the efficacy of specific models of outreach work, with emphasis being placed on the need to penetrate social networks and to contact those least likely to be reached by established services (ACMD, 1993). In this volume the natural history and aims and objectives of at least two advances on the traditional model of the professional outreach worker are described. The 'Indigenous Leader' model relies heavily on the life skills and experiences of ex-drug-users as health advocating outreach workers (see Chapter 12). The 'Peer Driven Intervention' all but removes the outreach worker by promoting a chain letter approach to risk reduction, one that is based on minimal engagement generating maximum numbers of contacts (see Chapter 13).

It is clearly important that we monitor and evaluate these various approaches and determine their relative efficacy (see Rhodes *et al.*, 1990; Kelly *et al.*, 1992). Yet such comparative evaluation should not be used to damn out of court community-based approaches that have value in specific contexts. It should not preclude matching particular styles of interventions (or combinations of interventions) to the aims and objectives of any given community-based initiative. Put simply, we need to be eclectic rather than proselytising in our approach to community-based interventions.

It is at this juncture that social research has a role to play over and above evaluation. By examining the nuances of behaviour and describing the drug patterns and profiles of drug using arenas and communities we can ensure that the intervention matches the target. For instance, it might be most appropriate to utilise the Indigenous Leader model to reinforce protective strategies amongst specific target groups of drug injectors. On the other hand, very specific health education information, such as the environmental risks to injectors of contracting hepatitis C, may best be disseminated through a peer-driven intervention. Alongside the management and coordination of innovative projects, outreach workers will always have a key role to play in ensuring that the appropriate technology is readily available to drug injectors and at drug using arenas. There are liable to be situations, for instance when targeting particular communities such as ethnic minorities, where a combination of all these approaches will be appropriate.

Notwithstanding these points, it is clear that risk and risk management is not simply an individualistic matter. These take place and are recreated in a social behavioural and interactive world. In that illicit drug use is largely a communal activity, so too should interventions operate at the level of social interaction. And just as social relations are fluid and subject to change, so too should community-based interventions be prepared to adapt and be flexible to shifting scenarios.

REFERENCES

Adams, J. (1995) *Risk*, London: UCL Press.
ACMD (Advisory Council on the Misuse of Drugs) (1993) *AIDS and Drug Misuse Update. Third Report*, London: HMSO.
Bean, P. and Wilkinson, C. (1988) 'Drug taking, crime and the illicit supply', *British Journal of Addiction*, 83: 533–539.
Beck, U. (1993) *Risk Society*, London: Sage.
Booth, R. and Wiebel, W. (1992) 'Effectiveness of reducing needle-related risks for HIV through indigenous outreach to injection drug users', *American Journal on Addictions*, 1: 277–287.
Burt, J. and Stimson, G. (1993) *Drug Injectors and HIV Risk Reduction: Strategies for Protection*, London: Health Education Authority.
Dolan, K., Stimson, G., and Donoghoe, M. (1993) 'Reductions in HIV risk behaviours and stable HIV prevalence in cohorts of syringe-exchange clients and other injectors in England', *Drug and Alcohol Review*, 12: 133–142.
Friedman, S. (1993) 'Going beyond education to mobilising subcultural change', *International Journal of Drug Policy*, 4: 91–95.
Friedman, S., Sterk, C., Sufian, M., Des Jarlais, D. C. and Stepherson, B. (1990) 'Reaching out to injecting drug users', in J. Strang and G. Stimson (eds) *AIDS and Drug Misuse*, London: Routledge, pp. 174–86.
Green, A., Pickering, H., Foster, R., Stimson, G. and Power, R. (1994) 'Who uses cocaine? Social profile of cocaine users', *Addiction Research*, 2: 135–226.
Grund, J. P., Blanken, P., Adriaans, N., Kaplan, C., Barendregt, C. and Meeuwsen, M. (1992) 'Reaching the hidden unreached: targeting hidden IDU populations with clean needles via unknown user groups', *Journal of Psychoactive Drugs*, 24: 41–47.
Johnson, B., Goldstein, P. and Preble, E. (1985) *Taking Care of the Business: the Economics of Crime by Heroin Abusers*, Lexington: Lexington Books.
Kelly, J., St. Lawrence, J. and Brasfield, T. (1992) 'Community AIDS/HIV risk reduction: the effects of endorsements by popular people in three cities', *American Journal of Public Health*, 80: 1483–1489.
McKeganey, N. and Barnard, M. (1992) *AIDS, Drugs and Sexual Risk*, Buckingham: Open University Press.
Murphy, S. and Waldorf, D. (1991) 'Kickin' down to the street doc: shooting galleries in the San Francisco Bay Area', *Contemporary Drug Problems*, 18: 9–29.
Ouellet, L., Jimenez, A., Johnson, W. and Wiebel, W. (1991) 'Shooting galleries and

HIV disease: variations in places for injecting illicit drugs', *Crime and Delinquency*, 7: 64–85.

Parker, H., Newcombe, R. and Bakx, K. (1987) 'The new heroin users: prevalence and characteristics in Wirral, Merseyside', *British Journal of Addiction*, 82: 147–157.

Power, R. (1994) 'Some methodological and practical implications of employing drug users as indigenous fieldworkers', in M. Boulton (ed.) *Challenge and Innovation: Methodological Advances in Social Research on HIV/AIDS*, London: Taylor & Francis. pp. 97–111.

Power, R. (1995) *Coping with Illicit Drug Use*, London: Tufnell Press.

Power, R., Hartnoll, R. and Daviaud, E. (1988) 'Drug injecting, AIDS and risk behaviour: potential for change and intervention strategies', *British Journal of Addiction*, 88: 649–654.

Power, R., Green, A., Foster, R. and Stimson, G. (1995) 'A qualitative study of the purchasing and distribution patterns of cocaine and crack users in England and Wales', *Addiction Research*, 2: 363–379.

Rhodes, T. (1993) 'Time for community change: what has outreach to offer?' *Addiction*, 88: 1317–1320.

Rhodes, F., Corby, N. and Wolitski, S. (1990) 'Risk behaviours and perceptions of AIDS among street injection drug users', *Journal of Drug Education*, 20: 271–288.

Wiebel, W. (1988) 'Combining ethnographic and epidemiological methods in targeted AIDS interventions: the Chicago model', in R. Battjes and R. Pickens (eds) *Needle Sharing among Intravenous Drug Abusers: National and International Perspectives*, Rockville, MD: NIDA, pp. 137–151.

Chapter 11

Heroin, risk and sexual safety

Some problems for interventions encouraging community change

Tim Rhodes and Alan Quirk

Most community interventions share an understanding that individualistic models of intervention are limited in their scope for achieving or sustaining behaviour change. It is recognised that HIV prevention interventions need to target more than individuals and individual behaviour change alone. This has led to the advocacy of social models of behaviour change among populations affected by HIV infection and AIDS.

Social models caution against the restrictive vision of individualistic models which tend to view health behaviour change as simply a product of an individual's perceptions, health beliefs and decision-making. They demand a more inclusive vision of change which encompasses both individual beliefs and behaviours and the factors which interact with these to influence the ways in which individuals think and behave. Interventions which conceive of individuals as the single or primary target and agent of change often exclude the possibility for facilitating concomitant changes in wider peer group and community norms about risk and health which help to mould, routinise and regulate individualised thinking and behaviour.

The common tendency to reduce 'behaviour change', and the factors which precipitate or influence such change, to the individualised unit of one is fast becoming outmoded by intervention models which target interconnected *groups* of individuals and social relationships as agents of change (Rhodes, 1993; Friedman *et al.*, 1992). Most of the chapters in this book share an understanding that individuals' attempts at behaviour change are often influenced by the ways in which *other* individuals think and behave. Interventions thus need to focus on changing the dynamics of how *groups* of individuals behave, and not simply on atomised individuals.

This chapter focuses on the problems and possibilities associated with sexual behaviour change among users of heroin. We begin by outlining the ways in which dominant research paradigms have studied 'risk' and 'risk behaviour'. Research definitions of 'risk' are discussed in the light of their implications for understanding how everyday norms influence the ways in which people perceive risk and act in response to risk. This then allows for an examination of how 'sexual risk' is perceived among heroin users and of how 'sexual norms' influence individual attempts at sexual behaviour change. This section of the chapter draws on ethnographic research undertaken in London by the authors.

The chapter closes with discussion on some of the key problems associated with norm-changing strategies designed to encourage sexual behaviour change among drug users. This discussion hopes to highlight some of the practical limitations associated with peer education and social diffusion interventions. It illustrates, for example, that many community-oriented interventions have an overly simplistic understanding of how social norms influence individual behaviours. It shows that while norm-changing strategies are needed in HIV prevention, they – like interventions oriented to individuals – may be only partially effective. The fact, for example, that individuals often *deviate* from norms often remains overlooked by interventions advocating community change.

In conclusion, the chapter cautions against the tendency for peer education and social diffusion interventions to be seen as a panacea to overcoming the limitations associated with individualistic interventions. The example of sexual behaviour change not only highlights some of the practical problems associated with norm- or group-changing strategies; it also questions the tendency to have an over-reliant 'faith' in these strategies.

NORMS, 'RISK' AND BEHAVIOUR CHANGE

Most research studies, particularly those of an epidemiological or quantitative slant, are unable to describe how risk behaviour is understood from the perspectives of drug users themselves (Rhodes, 1995). This means that epidemiological measures of 'risk' often fail to account for how 'risk behaviour' is perceived by those who engage in such behaviour. Without this understanding, such measures often fail to account for how risk perception and behaviour is influenced by the norms and routines of everyday lives.

Epidemiological constructions of 'risk'

The example of injecting drug use helps to illustrate this point. Contemporary research constructions of 'risk' associated with heroin use view 'risk behaviour' as inextricably bound up with the act of injection. It is probably fair to say that most epidemiological definitions of risk behaviour among heroin users are *synonymous* with injection. Injecting is *the* risk behaviour. This, understandably, is because of the HIV transmission risks associated with injection. The 'meaning' of injection for research and health promotion in the age of AIDS *is* the risk of HIV infection.

Yet qualitative and ethnographic research, which has aimed to describe how heroin users themselves view injection, points to the limitations of these dominant constructions of what 'risk' is as far as injecting is concerned.

When understood in the context of the norms, rites and rituals of everyday life, injecting may have very different meanings for heroin users than it does for researchers or interventionists. In the context of everyday drug injecting, the 'risks' which heroin users associate with injecting may have far less to do with the transmission of infectious disease (such as HIV or hepatitis) than with other risks or dangers which tend not to feature in contemporary measures of 'risk behaviour'. As our own qualitative research has shown (Figure 11.1), these include the risks of addiction and overdose, the risk of violence associated with dealing, buying and using drugs, the risk of damage to veins, and the health risks associated with making particular types of injection (e.g. when injecting into the groin) (Rhodes, 1995).

Qualitative research points to the importance of researching how the

---

Dependency
'If I don't have any sort of opiate I don't feel well and I can't function properly'

Overdose
'If you're injecting then obviously it's quite dangerous 'cos you could quite easily overdose'

Injecting damage
'It's inevitable I'm gonna end up losing an arm or a leg and I don't wanna do that'

Sharing injecting equipment
'Blood poisoning, hepatitis, HIV . . . I don't like the idea of anything going under my skin'

Using bad gear
'Buying bum gear . . . you could kill yourself . . . I'm just so dubious about street gear and what's in it'

Chasing/smoking
'I'm booting, can't be doing my lungs any good, my chest, it messes around with your body'

Buying
'The only way you can get it [money] is by ripping someone off'

Dealing
'We're really careful when we leave [dealers], sort of make sure we stash it somewhere'

General health
'It takes over . . . I mean even like eating properly'

Sexual health
'Heroin is the kiss of death to anyone's sex life'

Figure 11.1 Some risks associated with everyday heroin use

everyday routines of injecting behaviour influence how risk, and HIV risk, is perceived. The key point here is that behaviours which are, for public health reasons, considered 'risky' by the epidemiologist may be viewed as habitual, normal or mundane by those who engage in them. In addition, they may be seen to carry *different* meanings of 'risk'. Understanding how norms shape individual behaviours necessitates also understanding how norms shape perceptions of 'risk'. Appreciating what 'risk' and 'risk behaviour' actually mean to heroin users assists in developing practical responses to reducing risk specific to HIV and other infectious diseases. Without such an appreciation, we are more likely to fail in our endeavour to understand why it is that people behave as they do, and why it is that they continue to engage in behaviours which are known to carry a risk of HIV transmission.

It is therefore crucially important to recognise that the risks associated with HIV may be viewed by drug users as *relative* concerns (Rhodes, 1995). Without understanding the array of risks and dangers which heroin users themselves associate with injecting, it is extremely difficult to encourage HIV-related behaviour change. What health interventionists view as 'HIV transmission' behaviour may have alternative meanings for actors themselves. In the context of the everyday norms and meanings of injecting drug use, the risks specific to HIV infection may be given a far lower priority than many epidemiologists or interventionists could either imagine or wish for. This, as Margaret Connors has pointed out, is because the 'meaningful dimension' of the lives of drug injectors has 'been hidden behind an externally-constructed pastiche of risk behaviours only specific to AIDS' (Connors, 1992).

Risk intervention and risk reduction

These points on how social context influences risk perception have two key implications for the development of community interventions. First, it is naïve to expect individuals to make risk calculations or assessments in the way most models of health behaviour presume (Rhodes, 1995; Bloor, 1995). Individual perceptions of risk depend not simply on individuals' 'cognitions' and knowledge of transmission susceptibility but also on aspects of risk acceptability and priority (Douglas, 1986). As we show later in this chapter, perceptions of risk acceptability and priority tend to be a function of the norms and routines of lifestyle rather than of individual decision-making alone. At the outset, interventions need to recognise that risk perception is *socially* organised.

Second, the starting point for any risk reduction intervention is to understand how risk is perceived among those we wish to target. Working within dominant scientific constructs of what 'risk behaviour' is, interventions often have a restricted vision of what risk is for their target populations. As long as this is the case, drug interventions are left with what can only be described as glimmers of understanding about the social processes which influence how and why drug users behave as they do. These points illustrate the practical necessity of using qualitative and ethnographic research to develop future intervention responses.

QUALITATIVE RESEARCH ON HEROIN, RISK AND SEXUAL SAFETY

Ethnography and qualitative research is concerned with descriptions of how risk is 'lived' through everyday interaction and experience. The aim is to capture how risk perception and behaviour are organised by the norms and routines, chaos and unpredictability of everyday life. Such research stands in marked contrast to the technological order and predictability of scientific constructs of 'HIV risky lifestyle'.

Our qualitative research among heroin users in London aimed to investigate the sexual behaviour of heroin users, paying particular attention to the negotiation of sexual safety.[1] Two key tenets informed our research approach. First, we aimed to describe the *social meanings* heroin users attached to risk and risky behaviour. This allowed us to examine risk perception associated with behaviours known to carry a risk of HIV transmission (e.g. injecting and unprotected sex) as well as risk perception associated with behaviours which carried other dangers. Second, we aimed to better understand the *social processes* by which heroin users attached meaning to what they, and others, saw as risky behaviours. Taken together, the project not only aimed to describe *what* heroin users perceived to be risky, but *why* and *how*, on a day-to-day basis, certain behaviours were perceived to be more risky than others.

To achieve these aims, we undertook inductive interviews and observations with approximately sixty users of opiate drugs, the majority of whom used heroin. Those participating in the study included male and female injectors, chasers and snorters of heroin, the majority of whom used regularly or daily. We draw on this research so as to make some observations on the practical feasibility of interventions which aim to encourage 'community change'. Our research observations lend support to the argument that there is a need to develop interventions oriented towards norm- and group-mediated change. This, we believe, remains a necessary and under-utilised HIV prevention method among drug using populations. However, our research also points to problems in norm-changing strategies designed to encourage community change. This is particularly the case as far as sexual behaviour change is concerned.

SEXUAL RISK IN CONTEXT: PERCEPTIONS OF RISK SUSCEPTIBILITY

Almost all published surveys among injecting drug users indicate continued reductions in injecting risk behaviour, yet little or no evidence of sexual behaviour change. Such research has repeatedly shown that the majority of drug injectors are sexually active, that rates of partner change are relatively high and that there is a high degree of sexual mixing between injectors and non-injectors (Des Jarlais *et al.*, 1992; Rhodes and Stimson, 1996). Most importantly, surveys show that the majority of drug injectors report never using condoms with their primary partners, that a significant minority report never using condoms with their casual partners and that their reported levels of sexual risk behaviour are similar to those in non-using populations (Rhodes, 1994a). Researchers have got as far as exchanging *knowledge* about the fact that there is a considerable amount of unsafe sex going on but have made few attempts to systematically understand *why* sexual behaviour changes are so difficult or *how* such changes might be encouraged (Rhodes and Quirk, 1995).

Our qualitative research points to how HIV risks are seen by heroin users as relative concerns. We noted above that in the context of everyday injecting drug use, the HIV risks associated with injection may be seen to be less immediate or important than other risks, such as the risk of overdose, vein damage or addiction. For many drug users involved in the regular use and/or injection of opiates, the health risks associated with sexual behaviour were often viewed as less important than the health risks associated with drug use. As commented by a male injector of heroin: 'I haven't used condoms, that's where I think people slip up. They think about the works (needles/syringes) but they don't think about sex.' As another explained: 'I'm in a situation where I'm a drug user and don't wanna share needles and forget the sexual side and think you'll be OK.'

It is now a well-established observation that the social meanings attached by injectors to the act of equipment sharing have changed since the onset and awareness of HIV transmission. As commented by drug injectors: 'the only thing people used to worry about was getting hepatitis'. Prior to an awareness of HIV transmission, it was more likely that 'no one used to worry about any sort of disease' and that 'nobody used to think about things like that then'. Despite the emergence of 'post-AIDS' norms which make the sharing of used needles and syringes socially unacceptable as well as individually un- desirable ('I wouldn't dream of using anybody else's syringes'; 'it's really dangerous'), heroin injectors were more likely to 'take a chance' as far as sexual risk was concerned:

> I go out and get my syringes and they have a condom with them. But I can honestly say . . . that if it came to it and I was in bed, I could quite easily go along with it without a condom if the woman was in the same frame of mind . . . It's stupid.

Taking sexual risks or 'chances' was not seen to be particularly unusual, despite the fact that syringes were rarely shared. As was commented: 'We sleep together [unprotected] but I'd never share.' When any assessment of risk was made prior to, or during, sexual encounters, most heroin users were more likely to consider the potential for sexual and HIV risk in the light of their own or their partners' injecting practices than they were to consider them in the light of their own or their partners' sexual practices. As one injector said, when first meeting her current partner, she considered the likelihood of him having injected but 'didn't think about the sex' because she thought he 'was not much of a drug user':

> I know he's been around sexually but it was just the drugs I thought about. I mean he's got veins like bloody tree-trunks so I know he's never been that much into drugs.

A male injector also described how perceptions of HIV risk are largely dependent on an assessment of risk associated with drug use rather than sexual history:

> It's more of a drug thing. If you know that the woman uses a lot ... if she looks dirty, if she looks skinny and scrawny, if she looks like she doesn't look after herself. Like if she fixes a lot, then you'd think of yourself more at risk. If she's clean and healthy looking and she doesn't look as if she abuses herself, like banging up all the time, then you're more likely to think that she's alright.

This was also found to be the case among some non-injectors of heroin. A smoker of heroin, for example, indicated that: 'I wouldn't go to bed with any woman who was using intravenously without protection. End of story.' Another male non-injector remarked of injectors: 'She could beg and say "Look I'm clean and that" but, you know, I just wouldn't risk the temptation.' In this respect, heroin users' perceptions of risk susceptibility and their considerations about whether to use condoms were often made on the basis of whether sexual partners were known to be injecting: 'If I knew someone was using intravenously that would lower the chances of me sleeping with them'; 'knowing that she wasn't using intravenously just took away a lot of the doubt ... or even that element of me asking if she'd ever had an HIV test.' As was explained: 'There's no risk to us in the way we take our drugs ... or we'd have to think about using protection.'

These data illustrate how risk perception is a socially situated phenomenon. In the context of drug using and injecting lifestyles the HIV risks associated with injecting drug use have greater immediacy and priority for heroin users than the HIV risks associated with sexual behaviour. This is no great surprise. Individual assessments of risk which give greater priority to injecting drug use can be considered entirely *rational*. There *is* a closer proximity to HIV transmission risks associated with injecting than with sexual behaviour. This is not simply because of the relative transmissibility of HIV associated with sharing syringes and having unprotected sex, but is also a function of the ways in which perceptions of personal susceptibility and risk priority are socially situated. While for the health epidemiologist, sexual and injecting risks may be given equal priority in HIV prevention (both are HIV transmission behaviours), for the heroin user sexual risk is a *relative* concern, perceived in the context of other more immediate dangers.

SOCIAL/SEXUAL NORMS: PERCEPTIONS OF RISK ACCEPTABILITY

Individual perceptions of risk susceptibility are influenced by everyday understandings of 'risk acceptability'. What are considered 'acceptable' risks are to a large extent dependent on social context. This is what Mary Douglas means when noting that risk perception is socially organised:

> If a group of individuals ignore some manifest risks, it must be because their social network encourages them to do so. Their social interaction presumably does a large part of the perceptual coding on risks.
>
> (Douglas, 1986: 67)

What is perceived to be 'risk', and what is considered 'acceptable risk', are not static or necessarily shared by all individuals – be they drug users or epidemiologists – but are situated within different social contexts of meaning, belief and behaviour. Elsewhere we have used the example of overdose to demonstrate this point (Rhodes, 1995). Analyses of qualitative research have shown how overdose, and the risks and harms relating to overdose, have different meanings for heroin users than for non-users or other 'outsiders'. Our data shows how non-fatal as well as fatal overdose situations may be described by some heroin users with a degree of detachment which might not normally be the case when an acquaintance collapses on the sofa beside you. In the context of the routines of everyday heroin use, overdose is to some extent normalised and legitimised. Overdose can often fall within the boundaries of 'acceptable risks' associated with the injection of heroin.

Of key importance here is to note how the norms and routines of lifestyle shape perceptions of risk acceptability. Behaviours which carry with them health risks or dangers (whatever those risks may be) are often part of a wider structure or culture of behaviours common to everyday life. There is nothing unusual or spectacular about such behaviours from the perspectives of those who produce them, even if to outsiders they may seem somewhat bizarre or deviant. This sheds some light on the limitations of most conventional models of health behaviour in explaining risk perception and behaviour change. It illustrates, for example, that some risk behaviours need not be a product of individual decision-making or calculation about the costs and benefits of a specific action, but that these behaviours may simply be routine or habitual. The everyday norms regulating drug use and sexual behaviours highlight how risk is often a product of socialised habituation rather than individual choice or calculation (Bloor, 1995). These points are crucially important when understanding how social norms about sexual behaviour influence heroin users' perceptions of risk acceptability.

Our findings suggest that everyday norms encourage *safer* drug use yet *unsafe* sexual practices. The everyday normality and acceptability of unprotected sex in most heroin users' heterosexual relationships (particularly 'long-term' relationships) helps explain what are often seen to be 'anomalies' in drug users' reported risk behaviour. One such anomaly is that injectors may never or rarely share syringes, even with sexual partners, and yet will have unprotected sex, even with casual, and sometimes also HIV-positive, partners.

While it was common for heroin users to speak of not sharing injecting equipment as 'normal', it was conversely common for them to talk of unprotected sex as 'normal'. As one injector commented: 'It seems like more acceptable in a way to have unsafe sex than it does to share a needle.' Despite awareness that unprotected sex is HIV risky even if injecting equipment is not shared, unprotected sex was seen by many to be a common or normal feature of many heroin users' lives: 'It's normal for drug users . . . Nobody I know uses rubbers.'

But unprotected sex is a common feature of heterosexual relationships, whether or not either partner is a user of heroin. One of the most striking findings of survey research is that reported levels of condom use among drug users is almost identical to that among the heterosexual population in general (Rhodes, 1994a; Rhodes and Stimson, 1996). Perceptions that unprotected sex is 'normal' in heterosexual relationships are likely to be similar among drug users and non-drug-users. As we discuss later, not only does this point to some of the practical problems in encouraging sexual behaviour change, but it also questions the feasibility and appropriateness of norm-changing strategies among drug using populations. As one male heroin user said of unprotected sex:

> I should imagine everyone has done that [unprotected sex] whether they have used drugs or not. Everyone has taken a chance and had unprotected sex from whatever class you come from, from whether you use drugs or not. ·

In contrast to perceptions of what was acceptable risk in people's sexual behaviour, 'using works was just something that you never did'. Whereas unprotected sex was legitimised as a normal thing to do once an assessment of 'no risk' had been made, such an assessment was often not taken to alter the routines of injecting behaviours:

> I know he hasn't got AIDS and that, but I still wouldn't use them [needles/syringes]. Because there's always that risk

As described by another user of heroin who indicated that 'I can't see people changing their sexual habits' but who saw the sharing of needles as 'out of order' because 'there is no need':

When condoms are brought up, it's like 'Oh, yeah', they know we shouldn't do that, we should use a condom but we don't. When it comes to sharing a needle that is different. Everyone knows you don't share needles because there is no need. Condoms are different.

These data point to how social norms about sexual behaviour influence perceptions of risk acceptability as far as unprotected sex is concerned. Whereas social norms regulating drug use have to some extent encouraged and sustained community-wide changes away from injecting risk behaviour, social norms regulating what is appropriate or acceptable sexual behaviour tend to reinforce a status quo. This highlights the need for sexual norm-changing strategies to create the social environments where condoms are used as a matter of course. Community changes are required such that condom use becomes part of everyday normal and routine behaviour. Ideally, this would mean that condom use, like most everyday or routine behaviours, would become less a product of individual choice or calculation than a product of habitual behaviour; it would be something that is 'just done'. Where this is not possible, community changes need to create the social environments where individuals can, and do, exercise a 'choice' to use condoms. For these changes to occur, interventions need to encourage modifications in heroin users' normative beliefs about sexual risk acceptability as well as in the social meanings they commonly attach to unprotected sex.

SEXUAL NORMS AND ACCEPTABLE RISKS: EXERCISING 'CHOICE'

It is overly simplistic to say that social norms necessarily encourage unsafe sexual behaviour, and that because of this, unprotected sex is viewed as an 'acceptable risk'. While, in general, this may be the case, our findings also point to there being differential norms and expectations about sexual risk and safety in different social and situational contexts. This is equally true of the social norms which regulate injecting behaviour. What is considered by heroin users to be 'normal' behaviour is clearly context-dependent, and the norms and expectations which influence individuals' sexual interactions differ according to the specific social contexts in which they occur.

To illustrate this point we focus on how condom use results from interpersonal 'negotiation' in sexual encounters, which itself is influenced by individuals' perceptions of norms and expectations associated with sexual safety. This serves to demonstrate that risk-related action in sexual encounters is a function, not simply of 'individual choices', but of *negotiated actions*. Furthermore, we show that these interpersonal interactions, and the expectations that individuals bring to them, are influenced by socially organised norms regulating male and female sexual behaviour. Taken together, this shows how there is an interplay between the intentions of individuals, their interpersonal interactions and social/sexual norms which regulate communication and behaviour in (heterosexual) sexual encounters. While in practice most interventions are oriented towards change in individual behaviours, or, at best, at changing interpersonal interactions, they are most likely to be effective when they also target changes in social/ sexual norms.

Negotiating condom use: expectations and 'norms'

Our research pointed to how individuals' perceptions of norms regulating condom use differed by context. In commercial sexual encounters, for example, condom use was seen to have become the 'done thing'. As one female injector, who had worked as a prostitute for more than a decade, commented: 'before AIDS' many clients would seek to buy unprotected sex. However, there has since developed a norm or expectancy – among both sex workers and their clients – that condoms are used when having penetrative commercial sex. As she commented:

> It used to be quite hard getting them to use a Durex. Now they insist on it as well [although] you do get the odd client [who] will ask you for sex without a Durex.

She went on to add:

> Asking clients [to use condoms] is just one of those things. You just insist on it. I would say that ninety-nine girls [prostitutes] out of a hundred do insist on using a condom.

While in general our observations point towards sexual norms which encourage unsafe sex in non-commercial relationships – particularly those which are long term – this was not always the case. In certain contexts, it was likely for drug users to see condom use as a normal or expected feature of sexual encounters. This was most notable in male same-sex encounters, but also occured in some heterosexual encounters. As a gay man who used heroin occasionally said:

> It's different on the gay scene because it's the thing to do. It's always safer sex for me and for most of my friends it is. I probably don't know anyone that doesn't walk around with condoms in their pocket.

A norm or expectation that condoms will feature as part of first-time sexual encounters makes individual attempts to initiate or negotiate safer sex considerably easier. Such 'safety norms' help people to choose or 'do' condom use in two main ways. First, condom use can become a taken-for-granted, habitualised behaviour which is not perceived as something which needs to be 'chosen' or 'negotiated'. In these (ideal) contexts, condom use 'just happens'. Second, safety norms allow people to *communicate* to others that condom use is both normal and necessary, as 'something that I do all the time'. In short, individuals can *use* these safety norms in first-time encounters. As the comments of a female heroin injector illustrate:

> *[When you produced a condom . . . did you say put this on?]* 'Yeah, "Here you go" sort of thing – perfectly normal, natural.' *[So you gave the impression that it was something normal?]* 'Something that I do all the time, but unfortunately it's not!'

In contexts where safer sex has become the 'done thing', condom negotiation may often take a non-verbal form. An example of this is where the condom is passed from one partner to the other at the 'moment' when penetrative sex is to occur. Such a non-verbal action carries with it a clear request that the condom be used. At other times, condom negotiation may need only a 'perfunctory verbal exchange' between partners to ensure that condoms are used. As noted by a male chaser of heroin:

> I just said to her 'I suppose I'd better go and get, I'd better use something hadn't I?'. She's going 'Yeah'. And that's basically how it went.

These accounts show how a perceived 'norm' of condom use helps to endorse and reinforce individual intentions and attempts to use condoms. Where there exist 'safety norms', condom negotiation is made easier. When there exists a norm of non-condom use, negotiation can be far more problematic. Condom use has a different *meaning* in such contexts. Rather than a person's request for protected sex being perceived as something which is expected, 'normal' or 'rational', such requests may instead be taken as a charge of 'promiscuity'. As the comments of two heroin users show: 'If you insist on using a condom the other person gets the impression that you think they might be loose'; and 'It's basically saying she's a slag really and you should use a condom.'

The negative connotations that condoms may have in such contexts can lead to interactional difficulties, and even conflict or the threat of violence, if a request for protected sex is made:

> He just wouldn't discuss it. I mean he said, 'If you think that I'm some dirty so-and-so and that I've got AIDS' . . . It was impossible to talk to him. I mean, it'd be like trying to talk to someone who was insane.

This points to the observation that where there does not exist a norm or expectation that condoms will be used, there is likely to be a far higher level of ambiguity, uncertainty and delicacy about the timing, form and content of condom negotiation and the direction sexual encounters actually take (Quirk and Rhodes, 1995). In these situations, interviewees were not only aware that a request for protected sex might be 'taken the wrong way' and possibly heard as an 'insult', but they also knew that they might be asked to explain why condom use was necessary. This is a far cry from sexual encounters in which sexual partners share an understanding that condom use is the 'normal' and 'rationål' thing to do, where only a perfunctory verbal exchange or non-verbal communication is needed to make condom use happen.

The ways in which 'safety norms' influence interpersonal interactions and negotiations in sexual encounters have a direct bearing on the extent to which individuals are in a position to exercise 'choice' about whether or not condoms are used. Crucially, our findings suggest that there is a far greater need for interactional work when norms are broken, be these negotiations towards unprotected sex in situations where there exists a norm of condom use or negotiations towards protected sex in situations where there exists a norm of non-condom use. The implications of this for interventions are that people can, and do, deviate from safety norms. On the one hand, this points to the important (and often overlooked) fact that norm-changing strategies will only ever be partially effective: there will always be situations in which negotiated actions break the rules. On the other hand, this points to the importance of power in interpersonal interactions and in the ways in which safety is negotiated. Once again, this factor is often overlooked by norm-changing strategies, which tend to neglect the fact that safety norms may be broken in interactions where there exists a marked power imbalance in the ways action is negotiated.

Gendered risk: power in negotiated actions

The fundamental limitation of most prevention interventions is that they assume individuals are able to transform their 'choices' or 'decisions' about how best to behave into action. These choices are presumed to be made on the basis of individual assessments of risk or danger. In some contexts, individuals make choices based on how they perceive risk, yet their perceptions of risk are to a large extent socially organised. This means that there is no *single* rationality of what the right or 'healthy' choices are. Rather, there are 'situated' or plural rationalities of choice-making which are inextricably linked to the specific social contexts in which action occurs.

Neither are all choices equally available to all individuals. Choice, like risk, is a *relative* phenomenon. This leads us to make two observations about the limitations of individualistic models of prevention. First, the 'choices' which most models of prevention presume individuals to make are often a product of group decision-making and behaviour (see also Chapter 13). Second, individual and group choices are not necessarily equally distributed among all individuals or groups. Our example here shows how individual attempts to maximise sexual safety are constrained by the actions of other individuals, and how social norms about gender and sexual role have a bearing on individuals' relative power to exercise 'choice' in sexual encounters.

Unsafe sex may occur despite an individual's intention to use a condom and despite there existing a norm or expectancy that condoms will – or should – be used. Often unsafe sex is an outcome of negotiated decision-making between individuals where there is some form of agreement not to use condoms. The following description of condom negotiation by a male heroin user was offered as one such example:

> They've made me take it out of the packet . . . And I said 'Look, I don't want to, I hate these.' [And she said] 'OK, let's not use it.' Simple as that. And that's not once, that's [happened] a few times.

Yet unprotected sex was not always seen to have been consensually determined. Analyses of drug users' accounts of unprotected sex indicate that sexual risk varies not only by context but also by gender. It was far more likely for women to describe unprotected sex as having been the outcome of 'unequal' negotiations and as something over which they had little control. Unprotected sex was, in effect, seen to have been the *man's* choice'. Our data show that these unequal negotiations may range from non-physical persuasion to physical coercion. The following extract is from a female injector who, unaware of her own antibody status, was pressured into having unprotected sex by her HIV-positive partner:

> To him it was unnatural 'Why should we do it?'. And then there was the denial: 'They've made a mistake, it wasn't my blood test, I'm alright' . . . So there were a lot of arguments, a lot of tension.

As described by another female injector, who was also unaware of her own antibody status at the time, unprotected sex with her HIV-positive partner was often the outcome of unequal negotiations:

> I said, 'You've got to start using a condom, because the more risk you take in making love without safe sex, the more I've got the risk that I might die before you.' *[And what did he say?]* 'Oh, I'm sure they've made a mistake, I'm healthy, I haven't got nothing.'

The instances of unsafe sex between women and their HIV-positive partners are paralleled by other accounts which suggest that women and men often do not have equal power or control when negotiating safety in sexual encounters. Negotiating safer sex is not simply a product of carefully conducted interactional work between partners: in some situations no amount of verbal or non-verbal communication will make a difference. One woman gave a particularly clear example: 'He raped me . . . I asked if he wanted to [wear a condom] but obviously he didn't want to.' Constraints on women's attempts at condom negotiation were particularly evident when the initiation of protected sex was perceived to carry with it *greater* risks than unprotected sex. As the account of one female injector illustrates, the HIV risks of having unprotected sex may not outweigh the risks of suggesting that condoms be used:

I weren't allowed. [He] wouldn't let me go on about it . . . He'd go absolutely ape-shit . . . He wanted 50 million kids . . . He hadn't heard of contraception.

These extracts highlight that sexual risks are relative. In consensually determined unsafe encounters the perceived 'risks' or 'costs' of unprotected sex may not outweigh the perceived 'benefits' of enhanced sexual pleasure, displays of commitment, love, trust or permanency in relationships. In non-consensually determined unsafe encounters, there may be the addition of other perceived dangers associated with the initiation of protected sex, such as the threat or promise of sexual violence. As was commented, suggesting protected sex could mean that: 'He would not be happy. I'd get in trouble.'

In contrast to these accounts given by women, male drug users' accounts were more likely to indicate choice and control in heterosexual sexual encounters. The accounts of men with HIV-positive partners can be contrasted with those of the women in similar circumstances described above. Both men had female partners known to be HIV-positive and were unaware of their own antibody status (both later tested negative). However, both made what might be termed an 'informed choice' to continue having unprotected sex. The first said that he had not cared about sexual safety at that time because his 'relationship was more important than life itself'. The second 'went for two years unprotected' with his partner because he and his partner had wanted to have 'real sex':

Sometimes we decided to spoil ourselves and have real sex . . . We both decided to throw caution to the wind and have real sex for once, and we enjoyed it all the more although we both knew we were putting me at risk.

When viewed in context, it becomes clear that sexual safety is more than a matter of negotiation technique. What risk and safety actually *mean* to individuals differs depending upon the degree to which they have choice or control over the ways in which action is negotiated. For some of the women we interviewed it may be *rational* to opt for unprotected sex when other available options at the time appear to carry greater or more immediate dangers. For the HIV-negative male injectors having unprotected sex with their HIV-positive partners, such an action can be seen to be a product of a 'situated rationality' of informed choice-making where the specific meanings associated with unprotected (and unsafe) sex were perceived as more important than the risks of HIV. This position makes a considerable advance on 'single rationality' theories of risk which would posit that having unsafe sex with HIV-positive partners is a product of irrational behaviour where the 'wrong' choices are made (Rhodes, 1995).

But our point here is not simply that individual 'choices' about sexual safety are the product of 'negotiated actions' or that individuals' unsafe sex is sometimes the product of having 'no choice' in coerced sexual encounters. Rather, our point is that interpersonal communication between men and women in sexual encounters is itself influenced by wider gendered norms of inequality. It is less usual for women to have power and control in sexual encounters, as it is in many other areas of social life. The implication of these findings is that change is required not only in whether or not there is a norm or expectancy of condom use in sexual encounters but in whether or not there is a norm of *male*-oriented control or choice in encounters and relationships as a whole.

This is not to suggest that it is always or necessarily men who prefer unprotected sex. Our interviews with women also highlighted instances where women preferred unprotected sex and where persuasion or negotiation was necessary to coax their male partners round. This said, accounts suggest that it was more common for men to express a preference for non-condom use and more common for men to attempt to persuade women to have unprotected sex. These data suggest that interventions which encourage a norm of safer sex will assist individual attempts at condom negotiation, perhaps particularly among women. This, however, does not simply mean that individuals will necessarily conform to a norm of sexual safety. There will be situations, especially where there is a marked power imbalance in the way interactions are negotiated, in which individuals can exercise their choice to deviate from norms. Norm-changing strategies may encourage normative behaviour but they clearly do not guarantee 100 per cent success. Not only do our findings point to the normative importance of norm-breaking in people's everyday lives, but they also suggest that people's ability to exercise 'choice' in sexual encounters is unequally distributed by gender. Once again, this highlights the reality that norm-changing strategies may only be partially effective, particularly in encouraging changes in heterosexual sexual behaviour.

CHANGING 'SEXUAL NORMS': SOME PROBLEMS AND CONCLUSIONS

The six-million-dollar question for interventionists hoping to encourage sexual behaviour change among drug users is: 'If "sexual norms" can impede individual attempts at behaviour change, how do we change sexual norms?' This is a very 'big' question. Not only do we have to consider very carefully the question of how precisely 'sexual norms' influence individual behaviours; we need to consider whether and how such deep-seated 'norms' can change.

A key determining factor in creating the social conditions in which individuals can change their behaviour is social norms. While there is little evidence of sexual behaviour change among drug users and injectors, research has nonetheless found peer norms to influence sexual behaviour change among drug injectors and their sexual partners (Friedman *et al.*, 1991;

Abdul-Quader *et al.*, 1992). The everyday shared norms, values and practices common to a peer group, network or community – as our own qualitative research has shown – are important in influencing the extent to which individual behaviour changes can occur. This is primarily because individual actions are made easier when they conform rather than deviate from social rules. Deviating from group norms – or acting in socially unacceptable ways – is generally seen to be less desirable. Two observations can be drawn from our research on how norm-changing strategies might encourage safer sexual behaviour. These concern the dual aims of encouraging normalised condom use and encouraging individual 'choice' in sexual encounters.

Habituation

Where behaviours are routine or habitual it is often the case that no specific or explicit risk calculation is made (Bloor, 1995; Rhodes, 1995). Where behaviour is *normalised*, it is often unnecessary for individuals to step back and think twice about the risks or dangers associated with their actions. Everyday routine actions are *just done*. Their 'doing' does not require any prior thought or calculation and their consequences do not require any post-rationalisation or assessment.

This applies to behaviours deemed 'risky' as well as those deemed 'non-risky'. If to drug injectors the act of injection is a mundane and routinised behaviour, such action may be habitual rather than calculated. Injection may have become something akin to making breakfast or having a drink. The same may, and can, be true of safer injecting behaviours. If, for example, the cleaning of injecting equipment with bleach becomes routine it need not require individuals to make any explicit 'choice' or 'decision' about whether to use bleach. The same may hold true for condom use. If condom use in first-time heterosexual encounters is normalised – as it is in some contexts – there is less need for individuals to 'negotiate' or communicate about whether condoms will be used (they may instead have to negotiate non-condom use). This can be considered the ideal target for community change interventions: to normalise condom use as part of habitual actions where condom use 'just happens'.

Calculation and 'choice'

That habitual actions rarely require individuals to make calculated choices leads to our second point. This is that in the absence of interventions encouraging habitualised condom use, norm-changing strategies also need to create the situations where choices can be made. This may seem contradictory. On the one hand, we are saying that if condom use is habitualised, choices are not necessary, while on the other we are saying that 'choices' are a necessary part of condom use. It all depends on what the norms about condom use are. In contexts where condom use is something which is just done it may not be necessary to specifically negotiate or 'choose' condom use. But when there is a norm of non-condom use, individuals need to be in a position to exercise choice about whether condoms are used. In this latter scenario, condom use is likely to require some explicit negotiation or communication between partners since a norm or expectancy of non-condom use has to be broken before condoms are used.

This highlights what we consider to be an extremely important observation: where actions deviate from norms, choice or decision-making is required, yet when actions endorse or reproduce norms this is not necessarily the case. Because actions which conform to norms are considerably easier to make (they may not require any explicit negotiation), 'choice' only appears to be exercised when the norm is broken. Our data suggest that in contexts where condom use is the norm, a negotiated decision-making seems evident when making choices to have *unsafe* sex, whereas in contexts where condom use is not the norm, a negotiated decision-making is required when making choices to have *safer* sex. This underlines the rationale for changing sexual norms towards condom use since the more 'normal', routine or expected condom use is, the easier it is for individuals to effectively negotiate whether or not they have a choice about using condoms.

Some individuals may deviate from group norms

These points on habituation and choice-making lead to a conclusion which supports the need for changes in sexual norms about condom use. But not only do our data point to sexual norms about condom use being context-dependent (e.g. the prostitute who has safer sex with paying partners yet unsafe sex with non-paying partners), it also illustrates that individuals can, and do, deviate from group norms. This may happen, for example, when individuals negotiate unsafe sex in situations where both partners shared an expectancy of condom use. It is also the case in situations where individuals are unable to exercise choice about whether condoms are used, even despite the existence of norms supportive of condom use (e.g. where unsafe sex is coerced). This indicates that norm-changing strategies are not all-important. They, like individualistic interventions, may be only partially effective.

This applies not only where sexual behaviour is concerned. Whether or not syringes are shared provides an equally incisive example. While sharing, for example, may now be considered socially unacceptable or undesirable among injectors as a whole, individuals may deviate from this 'norm' in certain social situations. The potential for individuals to deviate from group norms is often overlooked by those advocating norm-changing strategies. We are not questioning the importance of changing sexual norms towards endorsing safer sexual behaviour. Rather, we are reiterating the importance of being realistic about the potential impact that norm-changing strategies can be expected to have.

Our data illustrate that it is certainly *easier* for individuals to conform to group norms than it is to break them. But the existence of 'healthy' group norms does not mean that all individuals will necessarily behave 'healthily'. While it is fundamental to recognise that individual choices and actions are socially organised, it is equally important to make the following two caveats when considering the potential impact of group- or norm-mediated changes. First, unsafe behaviour may be an act of individual volition. For example, in situations where there exists a norm of condom use, unsafe sex may occur as a result of coercion. Second, unsafe behaviour may occur through a process of 'negotiation' between partners. An example of this is where the act of unsafe sex or sharing syringes deviates from group norms yet is consensually determined between partners.

These caveats do not challenge the view that individual choices or actions are socially situated. Individual action is the outcome of the interactions of individuals in the context of their social environments. Yet if in certain circumstances individual actions can deviate from the norms of group behaviour, interventionists need to consider how far-reaching 'community change' can be. The ability of norm-changing strategies to change behaviour is obviously restricted to those within a peer group or community who 'choose' not to deviate from norms. While we do not expect norm-changing strategies to be any more effective or far reaching than this, these points are of particular relevance when considering the feasibility of changing sexual norms.

Can sexual norms be changed?

There is a danger that social interventions encouraging community change are seen as a panacea. A read of other chapters in this book highlights that there is little doubt of the need for such interventions. They are long awaited. They make considerable advances on most current models of prevention and behaviour change, which assume that individuals take action with little or no influence from other individuals or their situational and social context. At the outset, HIV prevention interventions often need to encourage changes in social norms and context so as to create the social conditions in which individual attempts at behaviour change become possible.

Not only do we know that group-mediated changes are possible among networks of drug users, we also know that changing peer norms about drug use can be a more effective way of creating and sustaining behaviour change than targeting and changing individual beliefs and behaviours alone (Friedman *et al.*, 1992; Rhodes, 1993). It is possible to conclude that despite the 'predatory' nature of some drug users' social relationships, there is also the possibility for endorsing or encouraging an interconnected system of peer support. Peer education and norm-changing strategies can work, at least as far as the changing of individual and group behaviours towards safer drug use is concerned (Fisher and Needle, 1993).

Research also points to the success that gay community-oriented inter-ventions have had in encouraging population changes towards safer sex (Kelly *et al.*, 1992; see also Chapter 6). But the aim and target of changing group norms towards safer sexual behaviour among heterosexual drug users seems a tall order. It appears to require a major piece of social engineering which cannot (and perhaps should not) be the function of harm reduction interventions. It is tempting to view the changing of sexual norms as an intractable problem. Harm reduction intervention has got as far as recognising the *importance* of sexual norms in influencing whether or not unsafe sex occurs and as far as advocating their change (Rhodes and Quirk, 1995). We have yet to debate, in any meaningful manner, *how* – or even if – this is possible.

Here we make two observations about the problems facing community-oriented interventions among drug users. These are: the nature of drug using networks may impede opportunities for collective change; and the nature of drug using networks may impede collective changes in sexual behaviour in particular.

Drug using networks and community change

To move beyond the strictures of interventions targeting individuals as agents of change, interventions first require a knowledge of the characteristics and structure of drug using networks. This is a prerequisite for understanding the possibilities for social diffusion of the 'processes by which an innovation is communicated through certain channels over time among the members of a social system' (Rogers, 1983: 5). So encouraging the social diffusion of intervention messages as a means of facilitating group-mediated change first requires an understanding of the 'contacts, ties and connections' between individuals in a social network (Scott, 1990).

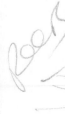

Once interventions have delineated the pre-existing channels of com-munication and influence within networks, it becomes possible to target these connections and relationships as agents of social diffusion and change. This is the underlying theoretical position of most peer education interventions. Borrowing from a mixture of social network analysis and social diffusion theory, peer interventions aim to encourage community changes both by targeting 'indigenous leaders' known to carry influence within a specific social group (see Chapters 6 and 12) and by exploiting pre-existing channels of communication and influence as they 'naturally occur' within social networks (see Chapter 13).

The principles underlying the social diffusion of community change are sound in theory (Rogers, 1983). However, in practice the nature of drug users' networks, and of the connections between individuals within such networks, may not necessarily be conducive to encouraging group-mediated change. It is clear that individuals are interconnected within a drug using network largely as a function of their drug use. The use, dealing, distribution and buying of drugs are greatly facilitated by having access to other drug users. While social relationships which emerge between individuals within these networks do, and can, encourage peer support, on the whole these networks are characterised by the functional needs and routines of the drug using lifestyle (Rhodes, 1994b; Power, 1995). It is perhaps for this reason that heroin users often talk of having 'acquaintances' rather than 'friends' within such networks, where connections with others come to have meaning through routinised drug use and not through other forms of communication or social interaction.

Our observations would suggest that the social relationships between individuals in drug using networks are generally characterised by a far higher degree of mistrust than the social relationships these individuals might have with others outside of these networks. This is not to say that smaller ego-centred 'support' and 'friendship' networks do not exist within larger drug using networks. Rather, it indicates that there often exists a culture of 'individualistic survival' within drug using networks which may impede attempts to encourage systems of collective support. Furthermore, it suggests that where a system of support or friendship exists it tends to be among a smaller subnetwork of individuals in the form of dyads or triads rather than among drug using networks as a whole.

However, it is important to recognise that this need not negate the possibilities for encouraging community or network support as far as drug use behaviours are concerned. Our research and observations also show that a system of peer support may exist even in the absence of 'friendship'. An incisive example is overdose. While overdose situations were sometimes characterised by inaction, where individuals neglected or ignored the fact that another user had overdosed, in general there existed a norm or expectation that drug users would help one another if overdose occurred (Rhodes, 1995). But community change interventions not only need to recognise the opportunities for encouraging collective or social change among drug users, they also need to recognise the limitations of these strategies. This is particularly the case when attempting to encourage sexual behaviour change.

Drug using networks and sexual behaviour change

The nature of social relationships within drug using networks may be conducive to encouraging a certain amount of peer support or collective change in drug use behaviours but this may not be the case with sexual behaviour. This is because the primacy of connections individuals have within drug using networks are a function of drug use rather than sexual behaviour.

What would be required for the diffusion of group changes on aspects of sexual behaviour is a sense of collective solidarity or shared interest associated with sexual as well as drug use behaviours. As social diffusion theory makes clear, the conditions necessary for community change and the likelihood of such change being adopted are closely linked to the facts that (a) the characteristics of communities govern the need and desire for change; and (b) the ownership of, and identification with, an intervention by a community governs the likelihood of it adopting and sustaining change (Rogers, 1983). In the absence of shared interest or connections based on sexual behaviour, it is unlikely that networks of drug users, *en masse*, will either desire or identify with each other concerning the need for sexual behaviour change in the same way as they might about changes in their drug use.

The 'master status' of drug using networks is that they are characterised by drug use (Rhodes, 1994b). The channels and content of communication within these networks are largely based on the shared knowledge and practices of drug use rather than those of sex and sexuality. Not only does the functionality of drug using networks often work against the creation of any meaningful sense of 'community', but our research points to there being little or no 'community' of interest on aspects of (non-commercial) sexual behaviour. It is fundamental to recognise that the notion of 'community' may be less of a social reality among drug using networks than among some other social groups, such as gay men, where there may be a shared sense of social and political identity and where infrastructures for action already exist (Patton, 1990).

The instability and transience of 'community identity' among networks of drug users introduces problems when attempting to foster 'community change' in shared norms and values. It means that 'community' potentially means less about the strength and meaning of social ties within drug using networks than it does about the mere fact that some social ties are there. Whereas among some gay networks, the strength of social ties is such that individuals self-identify as part of a socially as well as geographically or functionally bound 'community', it is far less likely that drug users see the nature of their network connections in these terms. In fact, it is far more likely for researchers and interventionists to view and speak about drug using networks as 'communities' than it is for the individuals within these groupings to do so themselves.

This makes the introduction of *group* sexual behaviour changes difficult. There may be no appropriate channels of communication or influence along which ideas of sexual responsibility and sexual behaviour change can diffuse. This gives important insights into why individual and group sexual behaviour changes are so difficult in comparison with changes in drug use behaviour. The key problem of initiating or encouraging sexual behaviour change among drug using networks is that the impetus or interest for such change is from *outside*. It has not been introduced, reinforced or endorsed from within drug using networks themselves. At the extreme there is something quite absurd and paradoxical about the idea of outside 'experts' introducing 'norms' into a 'community' to which they have no affiliation or membership. Yet this appears to be how community change interventions are approaching the problem of sexual behaviour change. It is precisely because sexual norms are part and parcel of everyday social life for all individuals, drug users or not, that the changing of sexual norms is so difficult within the restricted parameters of particular *sub*groups or *sub*cultures.

Sexual norms are made normative outside the parameters of drug using networks rather than within them. Individual sexual and gender identities take shape within wider realms of meaning and interaction on aspects of hetero-sexuality, homosexuality, femininity and masculinity. The targets and agents of change for encouraging changes in sexual norms, if the underlying principles of social diffusion theory are to be followed, are the communities of interest which shape and mediate sexual norms. These are not the same communities of interest as drug using networks.

These points highlight that to encourage changes in heterosexual sexual norms among drug using populations it may first be necessary to encourage changes in sexual norms among heterosexual populations as a whole. Such an intervention aim clearly surpasses the boundaries of most community HIV prevention initiatives. It is also questionable whether and how such deep-seated social and cultural values can be changed. While a great deal of social change has occurred in the past decade or so, sexual norms and inequalities are still very much reinforced by age-old conventional constructions of masculine and feminine sexual identity and gender role. This does not necessarily mean that changing sexual norms within drug using networks is an intractable problem but it does indicate that there are limitations to how effective community-oriented norm-changing strategies among drug users can be.

Concluding comment

There is a need for future HIV prevention interventions to target community changes towards encouraging a 'norm' of condom use. Our findings suggest, however, that there are limitations in the extent to which norm-changing strategies can achieve this, particularly among drug using populations. This points to some underlying problems in the theory and practice of community-oriented HIV prevention interventions among drug users.

If interventions are to understand better the interplay of individual and social action then it is wise for future ethnographic research not to neglect the question of precisely how 'social norms' influence individual behaviours. It is our contention that the problems associated with encouraging community-oriented changes in sexual behaviour highlight limitations in our current understanding not only of why individuals and groups behave as they do but also of how sexual norms can be changed. Interventions have got as far as advocating the importance of changing sexual norms but there have been few attempts to apply social diffusion methods to sexual behaviour change among drug using populations. This can be considered the next step towards minimising risk and maximising safety among community populations of drug users.

ACKNOWLEDGEMENTS

The data presented in this chapter are drawn from Department of Health-funded research which investigated the sexual behaviour and sexual safety of opiate and stimulant users. We also acknowledge the financial support of North Thames Region, which provides core funding to the Centre for Research on Drugs and Health Behaviour.

NOTE

1 This project was funded by the UK Department of Health as part of ongoing qualitative studies undertaken by the authors on risk perception among users of opiate and stimulant drugs. This chapter is based on fieldwork observations and interviews conducted between April 1993 and October 1994.

REFERENCES

Abdul-Quader, A. S., Tross, S., Friedman, S. R. et al. (1992) 'Peer influence and condom use by female sexual partners of injecting drug users in New York City', paper presented at Eighth International Conference on AIDS, Amsterdam.

Bloor, M. (1995) The Sociology of HIV Transmission, London: Sage.

Connors, M. (1992) 'Risk perception, risk taking and risk management among intravenous drug users: implications for AIDS prevention', Social Science and Medicine, 34(6): 591–601.

Des Jarlais, D. C., Friedman, S. R., Choopanya, K. et al. (1992) 'International epidemiology of HIV and AIDS among injecting drug users', AIDS, 6: 1053–1068.

Douglas, M. (1986) Risk Acceptability according to the Social Sciences, London: Routledge & Kegan Paul.

Fisher, D. G. and Needle, R. (1993) AIDS and Community-Based Drug Intervention Programs, New York: Harrington Park Press.

Friedman, S. R., Jose, B., Neaigus, A. et al. (1991) 'Peer mobilisation and widespread condom use by drug injectors', paper presented at Seventh International Conference on AIDS, Florence, Italy.

Friedman, S. R., Neaigus, A., Des Jarlais, D. C. et al. (1992) 'Social intervention against AIDS among injecting drug users', British Journal of Addiction, 87: 393–404.

Kelly, J. A., St Lawrence, J. S., Stevenson, L. Y. et al. (1992) 'Community AIDS/HIV risk reduction: the effects of endorsements by popular people in three cities', American Journal of Public Health, 80: 1483–1489.

Patton, C. (1990) Inventing AIDS, London: Routledge.

Power, R. (1995) Coping with Illicit Drug Use, London: Tufnell Press.

Quirk, A. and Rhodes, T. (1995) 'Condom negotiation among drug users', paper presented at Sixth International Conference on the Reduction of Drug Related Harm, Florence, Italy.

Rhodes, T. (1993) 'Time for community change: what has outreach to offer?', *Addiction*, 88: 1317–1320.

—— (1994a) *Risk, Intervention and Change: HIV Prevention and Drug Use*, London: Health Education Authority.

—— (1994b) 'Outreach, community change and community empowerment: contradictions for public health and health promotion', in P. Aggleton, P. Davies and G. Hart (eds) *AIDS: Foundations for the Future*, London: Taylor & Francis.

—— (1995) 'Theorising and researching "risk": notes on the social relations of risk in heroin users' lifestyles', in P. Aggleton, G. Hart and P. Davies (eds) *AIDS: Safety, Sexuality and Risk*, London: Taylor & Francis.

Rhodes, T. and Quirk, A. (1995) 'Where is the sex in harm reduction?', *International Journal of Drug Policy*, 6: 76–81.

Rhodes, T. and Stimson, G. V. (1996) 'Sex, drugs, intervention and research: from the individual to the social', *International Journal of the Addictions*, 31(3): 375–407.

Rogers, E. M. (1983) *Diffusion of Innovations*, third edition, New York: Free Press.

Scott, J. (1990) *Social Network Analysis*, London: Sage.

Chapter 12

Ethnographic contributions to AIDS intervention strategies

Wayne Wiebel

Ethnographic research has occupied a distinguished niche within the social sciences, dating back to the origins of both anthropology and sociology. As a consequence, the fact that ethnography has found a place within the applied research armamentarium mobilised to address the recent AIDS epidemic should come as no surprise. What has been unprecedented in the United States is the degree to which ethnography has been recognised as a key component in AIDS intervention research and service programmes. Nowhere has this been more prominent than in the US Public Health Service's initiatives to fund studies aimed at identifying effective strategies for reducing the spread of HIV among injection drug users (IDUs). Beginning with the National Institute on Drug Abuse's (NIDA) first major programme announcement for AIDS intervention demonstration research in 1987, and continuing through to their current Cooperative Agreement programme, ethnography has been an integral component of research designs (NIDA, 1987a, 1987b, 1990).

Two key factors influencing this development help to shed light on how ethnography came to play such a central role in US attempts to control the spread of HIV among drug injectors. The first was the established role ethnography had come to play within the field of drug research. The second was the lack of a solid foundation of knowledge upon which to formulate and test specific AIDS intervention strategies.

While by no means a dominant methodology in the field of drug research, ethnography had grown in recognition over the past few decades as a mode of scientific inquiry particularly well-adapted to contributing to our understanding of the social worlds of drug users and drug use. From the 1940s to the late 1960s, such studies are more notable for their findings and insights than for their number (Lindesmith, 1947; Becker, 1953; Finestone, 1957; Hughes, 1961). Since then, a notable increase in the number of published drug ethnographies reflects a growing interest in this focus of inquiry among trained ethnographers. There can be little doubt that the escalating prevalence of illicit drug use within the US, along with its perception as a major social problem, contributed substantially to this trend. Of at least equal importance was the growth in federal monies being allocated to support such research.

Following the creation of NIDA, Eleanor Carroll was foremost among a small cadre of project officers who actively encouraged the funding of ethnographic investigations. Readers interested in a more thorough discussion of the history of drug use ethnographies should refer to Waldorf (1980) and Ratner (1993).

By the late 1970s, interest in ethnographic drug research began to extend beyond individual studies to include a collaboration of investigators exploring the application of the methodology as a distinct mode of inquiry. A meeting of ethnographers was convened both to compile a collection of studies and to discuss prospects for future contributions (Weppner, 1977). This development was noteworthy in that it established the beginnings of a collective consciousness among ethnographers outside of academia. Ethnography's potential contributions were formally recognised to extend beyond scientific theory through applied research that could more directly influence public policy.

The first major opportunity to explore this potential was soon to follow. By 1978, phencyclidine (PCP) use was recognised to be widely prevalent across the US and was increasingly associated with bizarre adverse reactions. As the nation's primary drug abuse authority, NIDA was called upon for information and recommendations. Unfortunately, much of NIDA's drug use monitoring systems did not include a separate category for PCP and consequently were of little help in contributing to the limited body of current knowledge. Following in Eleanor Carroll's footsteps, George Beschner, NIDA's new principal proponent of ethnographic research, successfully commissioned a four-city ethnographic study of PCP users (Feldman et al., 1979). This work prompted a second meeting and volume of proceedings – this time including both ethnographers and policy makers in the drug field – to help establish a more direct link between ethnography and the policy arena (Atkins and Beschner, 1980). By the time AIDS and injection drug users emerged as a major public health problem, ethnography was well established within NIDA as a valued mode of scientific inquiry. In particular, its exploratory and descriptive capabilities to enlighten emergent trends and explain phenomena within the natural social context were widely recognised.

By the mid-1980s, a broad cross-section of US public health authorities were becoming increasingly involved in responses to address the AIDS epidemic. The Centers for Disease Control (CDC) played a leading role within the Public Health Service and, much to their credit, they recognised the need for involving other health authorities and were often instrumental in fostering such collaborations. In the case of NIDA, their established relations with the nation's publicly funded drug use treatment system together with their expertise in drug research suggested a natural role in pursuing the drugs and AIDS nexus. Amid growing criticism of inadequate action on the part of the government, a major appropriation of new funds for NIDA commenced in 1986 along with plans for a national AIDS demonstration research initiative targeting IDUs and their sexual partners.

NIDA appointed George Beschner to head up this substantial new undertaking. While the basic nature of the problem was clear, the specifics of what needed to be done and how best to do it were by no means apparent. It was known, for instance, that IDUs were spreading HIV through the sharing of injection paraphernalia. Yet the factors which influenced such sharing, the contexts in which such sharing took place, the meanings injectors associated with sharing, obstacles to the reduction of sharing, and effective strategies to discourage this practice were not well understood. Further, it was recognised that the vast majority of individuals at greatest risk – those not in drug treatment and still actively injecting in community settings – were not readily accessible through established systems of service delivery. Many detractors were openly sceptical about the potential of actively engaging IDUs in community settings and equally doubtful about their willingness or ability to alter high risk behaviour patterns. Given such formidable gaps in knowledge, not only was there a lack of consensus on the priority of research questions, but too often it was not even clear what were the right questions to ask.

Given Beschner's familiarity with the capabilities and strengths of ethnography, it is not surprising that he envisioned a role for this methodology within the demonstration research initiative, encouraging the inclusion of an ethnographer on the staff of proposed projects. Although the roles assumed by ethnographers varied widely between funded projects, in many instances they made substantial contributions to the successful implementation of the intervention demonstrations and made significant advancements in our knowledge of high risk behaviours. NIDA's National AIDS Demonstration Research (NADR) programme grew to include over sixty culturally and ethnically diverse communities across the US. By 1992, data had been collected on more than 43,000 IDUs and 10,000 sexual partners.

While all of the NADR projects made valuable contributions to our understanding of AIDS prevention among IDUs and their sexual partners (Brown and Beschner, 1993), two of the projects were selected as exemplary enhanced models worthy of being adapted in service oriented applications. These were the Indigenous Leader Outreach Intervention Model (Wiebel, 1988, 1993) and the Behavioural Counselling Model (Rhodes, 1993). These represented two different HIV prevention/intervention approaches examined by the NADR projects: the use of indigenous outreach workers who target social networks of IDUs in community settings and the use of a multi-session behavioural counselling strategy which can be incorporated into existing institutional settings. Recognising the importance of applying what had been learned from NADR as a part of service oriented initiatives, the Secretary of Health and Human Services legislatively mandated states to implement scientifically sound AIDS outreach intervention programmes with specific reference to the NADR proven models (Secretary of Health and Human Services, 1993).

THE INDIGENOUS LEADER OUTREACH INTERVENTION MODEL

The roots of the Indigenous Leader Outreach Intervention Model extend back to the late 1960s and the escalating interest in ethnographies of illicit drug use. Patrick Hughes, then a psychiatrist at the University of Chicago, pioneered a multi-method approach combining medical epidemiology and community ethnography to research and then intervene in neighbourhood outbreaks of heroin addiction (Hughes, 1977). Inspiration for this combined research and intervention strategy came from both sides of the Atlantic. The work of De Alarcon and colleagues in England (De Alarcon, 1969, De Alarcon and Rathod, 1968) fuelled his interest in studying the epidemiology of drug use. The work of Ed Preble in New York City (Preble and Casey, 1969; Preble and Miller, 1977) convinced him of the contribution ethnography could offer in understanding the social context of drug use. Later this combined approach was extended to include the study of adolescent multiple users in Chicago (Shick et al., 1978; Shick and Wiebel, 1981). Despite the success of this early work, by the late 1970s most of the key staff involved in these studies had left the University of Chicago, effectively curtailing further community-based investigations.

However, as AIDS began to spread among IDUs, lessons learned from Hughes' work in Chicago were not lost. If the approach had demonstrated success in monitoring and intervening in drug epidemics at the community level, might it not also hold promise as a research and intervention strategy targeting the spread of HIV among injectors? A small grant was submitted to CDC in 1985, resulting in the funding of a pilot project through the Chicago Department of Health. After little more than a year of promising though very preliminary results, a grant was received from NIDA as one of the first round of NADR projects, followed by a contract from NIDA to replicate the Chicago model in Baltimore, Denver, and El Paso.

Adapted to address the escalating public health threat of AIDS, what has become known as the Indigenous Leader Outreach Intervention Model merely incorporated HIV epidemiology within the framework of illicit drug epidemiology and ethnography established by Hughes. From a research standpoint, epidemiological analysis is critical to assessing the incidence and prevalence of HIV infection within high risk populations, monitoring epidemic progression over time, and evaluating intervention impact. From an intervention standpoint, epidemiology is crucial in determining the balance of intervention services required by different target populations at different stages of epidemic progression. For example, injector networks with relatively low rates of infection may offer a very high return on allocated prevention resources while having little use for treatment therapies appropriate for the AIDS-symptomatic patient. At the opposite extreme, an IDU network with a high rate of infection is very much in need of therapeutic intervention services while most appropriately requiring a shift in prevention resources to address the secondary spread of infection through sexual partners.

As applied to AIDS, ethnography's research role is primarily twofold. First, to document the norms, values and situational factors relating to HIV risk practices among targeted social networks. Second, to document changes in HIV risk practices over time and identify both obstacles and facilitators to such change. Ethnography's intervention role has expanded substantially from Hughes' earlier work and now includes a much more central direction over the implementation and evolution of intervention programming. Ethnographic contributions to the formulation and refinement of AIDS intervention strategies employed by the Indigenous Leader Outreach Intervention Model will be the focus of the remainder of this chapter. Readers interested in learning more about the outreach model can obtain copies of the intervention manual from the US Government Printing Office (Wiebel, 1993).

ETHNOGRAPHIC CONTRIBUTIONS TO AIDS INTERVENTION STRATEGIES

Ethnography differs from most modes of scientific inquiry in both the process of data collection and the analytic principles followed to generate findings. As a rule, an ethnographer does not adopt an *a priori* theoretical framework which assumes a pre-established relationship between variables to guide data collection or dictate a research design appropriate for the testing of a specific hypothesis. As a consequence, ethnographers are often able only to speculate in very general terms about the type of findings their research is likely to generate.

In the case of the NADR initiative discussed above, the general parameters of who and what the project's six ethnographers were to study was clear. Social networks of active injectors needed to be identified and then targeted for research and intervention. Through immersing themselves in the social world of injectors, establishing rapport and gaining the trust of subjects, the ethnographers laid the foundation necessary for ongoing data collection and analysis. In general, as data begin to accumulate around topics of research interest, ethnographers are increasingly able to understand how subjects interpret and make sense of their social milieu. As patterns emerge from the data, a continuing process of analytic induction begins with the postulation and testing of working hypotheses. Hypotheses are regularly revised to accommodate additional data until a best fit framework is found to explain the totality of the ethnographer's observations and experience. Often, emergent topics of investigation are identified that shift the focus of inquiry in unanticipated directions. Thus, a major strength of ethnographic research stems from its exploratory, flexible, and descriptive capabilities.

The examples of ethnographic findings which follow are neither intended outcomes nor serendipitous results of research activities. Ethnography was expected to yield valuable information, but the nature and implications of such findings could not be anticipated. Nor should the examples be considered as representative or typical of the ethnographic enterprise. Instead, they are the product of a number of ethnographers' evolving investigations and represent only a few of the many advances in understanding and insight that their work generated. The selection of these specific cases for discussion was based upon their diverse and unexpected contribution to knowledge of HIV transmission among IDUs together with the subsequent influence these findings had on refinements of intervention strategy.

All of the following examples attempt to highlight a number of factors found to influence high risk behaviours and the adoption of appropriate risk reduction measures. It is important to note, however, that the findings discussed are specific to the individual groups and social contexts under investigation. Interventionists interested in learning from these experiences may benefit from an analysis of similar influences within their own target populations, but would be ill-advised to independently adjust their own intervention strategies based on these findings alone.

Social organisation and promotion of risk reduction

The social networks of IDUs targeted for intervention by the outreach model consist of groups of individuals who regularly interact with each other based upon their reciprocal needs to obtain and inject drugs. Through establishing affiliations within IDU networks, injectors are able to procure drugs and injection paraphernalia, access places to inject, form partnerships to obtain the money required to supply their drug habits, and obtain information which may prove useful to them.

Because injectors rarely possess the resources to purchase large quantities of drugs, most regularly frequent dealers at public 'copping areas', private 'house connects', or 'shooting galleries' where drugs are sold as well as injected. Given their central role as congregation areas where large numbers of injectors cross paths, they are focal points both for the deployment of outreach activities and for ethnographic inquiry.

Reyes Ramos, the ethnographer for the El Paso, Texas, project, was introduced to the city's most active street drug scene by an outreach worker who was a former heroin addict with long-standing, high-status relations within this IDU social network.[1] Over the course of his observations and interviews with members of this target population, Ramos noted what seemed to be an extraordinary influence of enforcement authorities on the distribution and use of illicit drugs (Ramos, 1989).

Similar to most inner-city communities with high concentrations of drug addicts, this area was subject to heavy police patrolling. However, because the neighbourhood, or *barrio*, was directly across the major border crossing from Mexico, there was an additional, intensive presence of border patrol agents. Given the fact that it was difficult to distinguish the nationality of most injectors within this network, the probability of being stopped and interrogated was disproportionately high. As a consequence, addicts sought to minimise the amount of time they were in possession of narcotics and injection paraphernalia. In adapting to this situation, the social organisation of drug distribution and the drug taking practices of injectors exemplified a number of accommodations to lessen the risk of arrest. Each drug dealer was accompanied by one or more lower-status addicts, disparagingly referred to as *cucarachos*, who rented out injection equipment. These teams regularly moved about the *barrio* in an attempt to minimise the risk of attracting attention. When users and dealers connected, addicts typically bought drugs, rented injection paraphernalia, injected in a nearby site out of public view, and exited as quickly as possible.

In recognising these patterns, identifying the roles and motivations of participants, and determining the factors that influenced them, the ethnographer was able to assess the limitations of some standard risk reduction strategies. That is, suggestions that IDUs not share needles or that they attempt to disinfect used injection equipment were not likely to achieve high rates of compliance as long as addicts were not willing to carry anything illicit (drugs or syringes) or potentially incriminating (bleach). Further, it was not the addict who exercised the greatest control over the potential infectiousness of equipment used for injection. It was the relatively low-status renter of the equipment required for injection who was most influential in determining the circulation rate of potentially infective supplies in the rental market.

As a result of this analysis, it was decided that a specific strategy targeting injection equipment renters should be developed. Given the underlying economic nature of such exchanges and the desire of renters to maximise their proceeds from the business, a marketing perspective was integrated into the prevention campaign developed to target renters. Following education on the dangers of HIV transmission through the sharing of injection paraphernalia, renters were instructed in bleach decontamination procedures which were to be used when new sterile supplies were not available. It was then suggested that the marketing of new or used rental equipment as sterile or properly decontaminated[2] might increase the demand for their goods and enhance their reputation as someone who cares about the well-being of 'clients'. Alternatively, as expectations of the availability of safe injection equipment grew, there was the possibility that they might lose business should clients suspect that their goods were potentially infective. Provision to make free bleach available to renters was made along with ongoing reinforcement of AIDS prevention messages to all segments of the targeted population.

Identification of high risk practices through direct observation

One of the primary research roles of ethnography within our intervention design is to document norms, values, and situational factors relating to high risk behaviour. Through the direct observation of drug injecting practices, a number of previously unexplored high risk behaviours were brought to attention.

On a visit to a shooting gallery on a site visit to the El Paso project, addicts were witnessed unknowingly engaging in a high risk practice while otherwise attempting to comply with standard risk reduction procedures. The following day, it was learned that Steve Koester, the Denver ethnographer, had independently observed similar behaviour patterns in Denver, leading to identical concerns about the adequacy of existing AIDS prevention education. What had been witnessed was injectors first flushing previously used syringes with water and then bleach as a disinfectant measure. They would then draw up more water from the same shared communal container to rinse out residual bleach and then again to dissolve their drugs into an injectable solution. At issue was the fact that everyone frequenting the gallery was using the same shared container of water both to liquefy their drugs prior to injection and then to rinse out the syringe after injection to prevent the needle from clogging with dried blood. After extended periods of use, the water remaining in such containers became visibly tainted by the small amounts of blood left by previous users.

Koester also observed that IDUs attempting to reduce HIV risk through the bleaching of shared syringes were unwittingly continuing to place themselves at risk through the sharing of 'cookers' used to heat solutions for injection and 'cottons' used to filter these solutions when being drawn up into the syringe (Koester et al., 1990; see also Chapter 9 of this book).

In response to this emerging evidence, outreach workers were briefed and encouraged to spread the word about these potential sources of HIV transmission along with risk reduction options for avoiding them. Because ethnographic evidence also suggested that it was often difficult for injectors to access a supply of fresh water, small containers of sterile water were added to the prevention materials regularly distributed by outreach staff. Through word of mouth and on the labels of bottled water, IDUs were cautioned against sharing the contents with anyone else.

Shooting galleries and HIV transmission

As studies of HIV transmission among IDUs began to accumulate, an association was noted between the use of shooting galleries by injectors and increased risk of HIV infection (Marmor et al., 1987). While such an association was not always found (Watters, 1989), common sense suggested that as these were places where numerous injectors congregated to use drugs, sharing would often take place. Thus, shooting galleries at least posed a substantial risk as epicentres of HIV transmission.

In order to increase understanding of the nature of this potential risk and the relationship between gallery attendance and the spread of HIV, the Chicago ethnographic team of Larry Ouellet, Antonio Jimenez, and Wendell Johnson commenced an exploratory investigation. Each ethnographer supervised an AIDS outreach team in different community areas and was familiar with local IDU social networks. Areas of inquiry included users' definitions of what constituted a shooting gallery, factors influencing the use of galleries, and behaviour patterns associated with their use (Ouellet et al., 1991).

Analysis revealed three distinct types of place frequented by IDUs for the primary purpose of taking drugs. Interestingly, not all of these were considered to be shooting galleries by the target population. Some groups considered shooting galleries to include any place where addicts could go to inject, but others used more specific criteria in their definitions so as to include, for example, only places run as a business operation. For purposes of developing the present typology, the most general classification scheme of what constituted a shooting gallery was utilised.

The first identified category, 'the cash gallery', is run like a business. A fee is typically charged for admission and one or more individuals are responsible for the gallery's operation. In addition to offering a place to inject, such establishments may provide related services including the sale of drugs, the sale or rental of syringes, and a 'house doctor' who will inject clients for a fee. Almost all commercial galleries have a formal set of rules which clients are expected to adhere to. Operators make sure clients are aware of these rules and enforce compliance.

The second type of place IDUs frequent to inject drugs is the 'taste gallery'. Taste galleries are noteworthy in that they are operated out of an addict's room or apartment for the benefit of acquaintances in need of a desirable place to inject. The difference between a cash gallery and a taste gallery may be likened to the difference between going to a restaurant or a friend's house to eat. Not just anyone can show up at a taste gallery and expect to be welcomed. Further, reciprocity at taste galleries is not so formal as is the case in a commercial exchange although, whether explicitly set forth or not, some form of exchange is expected in return for the hospitality provided. Most often, the expectation is that the occupant will receive a small portion, or taste, of the drugs the acquaintance has brought to inject. In addition to the sharing of their room, residents may also offer visitors the paraphernalia needed to inject.

The third category of shooting gallery is called the 'free gallery' because no expense is associated with its use. Free galleries are often found in abandoned buildings but also include a wide variety of other places which offer relative privacy including alleys, public rest-rooms, and secluded areas within public parks. One characteristic common to many free galleries is a lack of available running water. As a consequence, containers of water are brought in and left at the site for the convenience of others who will visit later.

Within the communities which had been the focus of the ongoing AIDS intervention activities were found these three types of shooting gallery which represented a range in the potential for transmitting HIV. At one extreme were the cash galleries which tended to be very receptive to outreach and regularly accepted AIDS prevention materials including bleach, 'sharps containers' for syringe disposal, water, alcohol wipes, literature, and the like. Further, cash gallery operators tended to willingly assume the role of AIDS prevention advocacy and integrate risk reduction measures into the rules of the house.

At the other extreme, taste and free galleries represented a greater intervention challenge. Taste galleries, though among the most often frequented by the subjects, were difficult to identify and gain access to. Contributing to these difficulties was the fact that many injectors did not think of these more restricted sites as galleries and the individuals who ran such operations were hesitant to acknowledge the fact because they did not want to become known as gallery operators outside of the small, private networks who were allowed entry. Free galleries, on the other hand, had no one in charge to advocate AIDS prevention or enforce hygienic injection practices. Further, a lack of running water and a proliferation of disposed or hidden syringes greatly increased the risk of water and other injection equipment being shared. In the case of hidden or 'stashed' syringes, owners would probably be unaware that another injector might have found, used, and replaced the syringe. As a consequence, such IDUS might report and believe that they had stopped sharing needles when in fact this was not the case.

Findings from this investigation emphasised the need to continue targeting cash shooting galleries to reinforce AIDS prevention advocacy among operators and maintain adequate supplies of prevention materials. A recognition of the problems posed by taste and free galleries led to the development of new intervention strategies. The campaign to educate IDUs about the risk of sharing water and other injection equipment was modified to include issues specific to taste and free galleries. Outreach workers talked to clients about the risks identified in gallery-like places where numbers of friends went to inject together. Clients were encouraged to make supplies of prevention materials available at such places and to promote the adoption of risk reduction measures among the injectors who frequented these private premises. Individuals who frequented free galleries were urged to carry the one-ounce bottles of bleach and water outreach workers distribute in order to decontaminate previously used equipment and avoid the sharing of communal water. Outreach staff further sought to identify all free galleries in their communities and keep them regularly supplied with bottles of bleach and water for individual use.

Interpretation of AIDS prevention messages

AIDS outreach prevention activities are guided by five primary objectives. These are to increase AIDS awareness; to encourage individual risk assessment; to suggest a broad range of viable risk reduction alternatives; to reinforce risk reduction messages; and to promote prevention advocacy.

In encouraging the adoption of risk reduction measures to address blood-borne transmission among IDUs, projects rely upon a hierarchical framework to help convey the relative risk of alternative measures. These range from the most effective, to stop injecting or to stop the sharing of injection equipment, to less effective practices such as always using bleach to decontaminate shared paraphernalia, increasing the use of bleach when sharing, or reducing the frequency of sharing and the number of sharing partners.

Following San Francisco's lead, the Chicago outreach projects adopted bleach distribution as one practical risk reduction alternative in situations where a sterile syringe is not available or the sharing of a previously used syringe cannot be avoided (Newmeyer, 1988). Experience had taught us that, irrespective of intention or degree of motivation to adopt a risk reduction strategy, injectors could be expected to maintain compliance only when the means to accomplish a risk reduction measure were readily available. Hence, IDU social networks were flooded with one-ounce bottles of bleach and this strategy was found to be very well-received by target populations, giving little cause for concern that this approach was anything other than a success. Clearly, getting off drugs or not sharing injection equipment at all are preferable risk reduction measures which many clients did choose to adopt, but for the remainder, bleach decontamination procedures appeared to be a well-accepted option.

However, some doubts soon arose. The cause prompting a re-evaluation of this prevention strategy came from the most unfortunate and disturbing experience of an IDU subject with whom one ethnographer, Larry Ouellet, had established close and trusting ties. The subject sought out Ouellet to talk about an issue he was quite anxious about. In their conversation, the subject revealed that he was concerned about having possibly contracted HIV. The previous evening he had visited a friend and, while there, the friend offered to share a bag of cocaine with him. Unfortunately, he was not carrying his own syringe or bleach at the time. Larry asked why he hadn't gone out to get either a syringe or bleach. The subject said that he had considered the possibility but was convinced that, should he leave, by the time he returned there would be no cocaine left to inject. As a consequence, with great turmoil, he took the just-used syringe from someone he knew to be HIV positive and injected his share of the remaining cocaine.

While the possible tragic outcome of this event is quite obvious, those familiar with the compulsive drives associated with chemical dependence will not find the subject's seemingly irrational decision surprising. As a case-study contributing to ethnographic analysis of compliance with risk reduction measures, the new data had a profound influence on the understanding of how prevention messages were being interpreted. By distributing bleach and encouraging bleach disinfection procedures, this seemingly successful prevention strategy had been inadvertently interpreted by target audiences in a way that precluded the consideration of other potential decontaminants.

Had the client thought about other options to decontaminate or at least flush out residual HIV from the syringe, such as using vinegar, alcohol, mouthwash, or even soapy water, it would have been far better than taking the syringe just used by someone else and sticking it directly into his vein. Of course, such measures would not guarantee prevention of infection but at least they would reduce this risk and minimise the quantity of any active virus transmitted.

In response to this finding, outreach staff were informed and risk reduction messages relating to bleach distribution were modified. Instead of merely promoting bleach disinfection, clients were educated in the importance of attempting to disinfect or at least thoroughly clean any previously used injection equipment. The thrust of this prevention strategy thus shifted from bleach as a disinfectant to disinfection, with bleach being one of the most effective but by no means the only rinsing agent available to them.

CONCLUSION

The inclusion of an ethnographic component within AIDS intervention research and service initiatives holds potential for significant enhancements to project capabilities. While hopefully instructive, the preceding examples can only serve to suggest the types of contribution ethnography can provide. It is furthermore important to note that other types of methodologies do not lend themselves to the types of findings that are the mainstay of ethnographic research.

Yet, ethnography is by no means a panacea for effective interventions or a solution to the shortcomings of existing interventions that have been implemented without it. As a very labour-intensive and time-consuming methodology, it is best integrated within and implemented in conjunction with a planned intervention. Any attempt to plug an ethnographer into a troubled project as a 'quick fix' is almost certain to result in disappointment and failure. Neither should the employment of an ethnographer be considered to ensure the types of practical benefits suggested in this chapter. Irrespective of training, an ethnographer may not prove successful in establishing rapport with target populations or in developing positive working relations with other intervention staff.

Furthermore, forging a productive working relationship with ethnographers is not always an easy task for project leadership staff. Perhaps due to tradition within the discipline and natural selection in the choosing of a career, many ethnographers prefer to work independently. Also, by virtue of their analytic induction framework, they tend to be more interested in developing their own working hypotheses than in helping to test the *a priori* hypotheses of quantitatively oriented colleagues. Such characteristics in no way preclude the possibility of successfully integrating ethnographers within a multi-disciplinary team, but they do suggest that understandings and expectations are best worked out initially and not after problems develop. All scientific methodologies have both strengths and limitations which ultimately define their appropriate application and analytic potentialities. For a multi-disciplinary team to make the most of its constituent parts and avoid unrealistic expectations, a formal agreement of roles and responsibilities should be reached for all planned activities and work products.

It would seem that applications for ethnography within AIDS and other community-based interventions are beginning to be realised. One unfortunate consequence of the growing market for trained professionals is that the demand for ethnographers has begun to exceed the pool of available candidates. Nowhere is this more apparent than in the need for experienced minority researchers. It is certainly not necessary to match the race or ethnicity of ethnographers with that of their subjects, and some would argue that such differences often contribute to insights which might otherwise be overlooked. Yet it is difficult to deny that current and future understandings of topics studied by ethnographers would be greatly enhanced by a larger representation of minorities contributing to that body of knowledge.

For this to happen in the foreseeable future a number of changes must take place within schools of higher education. Most importantly, courses in qualitative methods and support for students wishing to undertake ethnographic work must be expanded. A bias currently exists in many academic social science departments favouring theory-based studies over applied research. One means of countering this obstacle may be to expand ethnographic training opportunities within graduate schools with applied orientations such as public health, urban studies, public policy administration, social work, nursing, and the like. Finally, these graduate programmes must be able to attract capable and enthusiastic candidates. Recognition of the work of current ethnographers can only help in this regard, as would the continued availability of well-paying positions in the job market.

NOTES

1 The intervention model refers to such outreach workers as indigenous leaders. In the argot of the Mexican/American drug scene, high-status addicts, such as Pete who is used in this example, are referred to as *tecato bueno*.
2 Recent research has suggested that contaminated injection equipment must be exposed to full-strength bleach for at least thirty seconds in order to inactivate residual HIV (Shapshak *et al.*, 1993) and that many injectors who use bleach in an attempt to disinfect syringes do not always meet this criterion (Gleghorn *et al.*,

1994). At the time of this study, the bleaching protocol called for syringes to be filled and flushed with full-strength bleach twice and then thoroughly rinsed twice with water before using. Given what is now known, this may not always have resulted in complete decontamination but it did provide a viable risk reduction (if not prevention) alternative.

REFERENCES

Akins, C. and Beschner, G. (eds) (1980) *Ethnography: A Research Tool for Policymakers in the Drug and Alcohol Fields*, US Department of Health and Human Services Publication No.(ADM) 80–946.

Becker, H.S. (1953) 'Becoming a marijuana user', *American Journal of Sociology*, 59: 235–242.

Brown, B. and Beschner, G. (eds) (1993) *Handbook on Risk of AIDS: Injection Drug Users and Sexual Partners*, Westport, CT: Greenwood Press.

De Alarcon, R. (1969) 'The spread of heroin abuse in a community', *Bulletin on Narcotics* 12: 17–22.

De Alarcon, R. and Rathod, R. (1968) 'Prevalence and early detection of heroin abuse', *British Medical Journal* 2: 533–549.

Feldman, H., Agar, M. and Beschner, G. (eds) (1979) *Angel Dust: An Ethnographic Study of PCP Users*, Lexington, MA: DC Health/Lexington Books.

Finestone, H. (1957) 'Cats, kicks and color', *Social Problems*, 5: 3–13.

Gleghorn, A.A., Doherty, M.C., Vlhaov, D., Celentano D.D. and Jones, T.S. (1994) 'Inadequate bleach contact times during syringe cleaning among injection drug users', *Journal of Acquired Immune Deficiency Syndromes*, 7(7): 767–772.

Hughes, H.M. (1961) *The Fantastic Lodge: The Autobiography of a Drug Addict*, New York: Fawcett World Library.

Hughes, P. (1977) *Behind the Wall of Respect: Community Experiments in Heroin Addiction Control*, Chicago: University of Chicago Press.

Koester, S., Booth, R. and Wiebel, W. (1990) 'The risk of HIV transmission from sharing water, drug mixing containers and cotton filters among intravenous drug users', *International Journal on Drug Policy*, 1(6): 28–30.

Lindesmith, A. (1947) *Opiate Addiction*, Bloomington, IN: Principia Press.

Marmor, M., Des Jarlais, D. C., Cohen, H., Friedman, S., Beatrice, S., Dubin, N. *et al.* (1987) 'Risk factors for infection with HIV among intravenous drug abusers in New York City', *AIDS*, 1: 39–44.

Newmeyer, J. (1988) 'Development of a strategy to combat HIV contagion among San Francisco intravenous drug users', in R. Battjes and R. Pickens (eds) *Needle Sharing among Intravenous Drug Abusers: National and International Perspectives*, National Institute on Drug Abuse Research Monograph 80, Washington DC: Department of Health and Human Services Publication No. (ADM) 88–1567.

—— (1987a) Program Announcement DA-87–13, 'AIDS community Outreach Demonstration Project'.

—— (1987b) Request for Proposal 271–87–8208, 'Indigenous Leader Outreach to IV Drug Abusers'.

NIDA (National Institute on Drug Abuse) (1990) Program Announcement DA–90–02, 'A Cooperative Agreement for AIDS Community-Based Outreach/Intervention Research'.

Ouellet, L., Jimenez, A., and Johnson, W. (1991) 'Shooting galleries and HIV disease: variations in places for injecting illicit drugs', *Crime and Delinquency*, 37(1): 64–85.

Preble, E. and Casey, J. (1969) 'Taking care of business: the heroin user's life on the street', *International Journal of the Addictions*, 4:1–24.

Preble, E. and Miller, T. (1977) 'Methadone, wine and welfare', in R. Weppner (ed.) *Street Ethnography*, Beverly Hills: Sage Publications.

Ramos, R. (1989) 'To be in the fire: drug trends in El Paso, Texas', in *Community Epidemiology Work Group: Epidemiologic Trends in Drug Abuse, Proceedings June 1989*, US Government Printing Office 248–963:00768.

Ratner, M. (1993) 'The role of ethnography in understanding and preventing drug abuse', report to the Office of Technology Assessment, US Congress, Washington, DC.

Rhodes, F. (1993) *The Behavioural Counseling Model for Injection Drug Users: Intervention Manual*, Washington, DC: National Institutes of Health Publication No. 93–3579.

Secretary of Health and Human Services (1993) *Federal Register* 58, 60:17064.

Shapshak, P., McCoy, C., Rivers, J., Chitwood, D., Mash, D., Weatherby, N. *et al.* (1993) 'Inactivation of HIV–1 at short time intervals using undiluted bleach', *Journal of Acquired Immune Deficiency Syndromes*, 6: 218–219.

Shick, J. and Wiebel, W. (1981) 'Congregation sites for youthful multiple drug abusers: locations for epidemiological research and intervention', *Drug and Alcohol Dependence*, 7: 63–79.

Shick, J., Dorus, W. and Hughes, P. (1978) 'Adolescent drug using groups in Chicago parks', *Drug and Alcohol Dependence*, 3: 199–210.

Waldorf, D. (1980) 'A brief history of illicit-drug ethnographies', in C. Akins and G. Beschner (eds) *Ethnography: A Research Tool for Policymakers in the Drug and Alcohol Fields*, US Department of Health and Human Services Publication No. (ADM) 80–946.

Watters, J. (1989) 'Observations on the importance of social context in HIV transmission among intravenous drug users', *Journal of Drug Issues*, 19(4): 9–26.

Weppner, R. S. (ed.) (1977) *Street Ethnography*, Beverly Hills: Sage Publications.

Wiebel, W. (1988) 'Combining ethnographic and epidemiologic methods in targeted AIDS interventions: the Chicago model', in R. Batyjes and R. Pickens (eds) *Needle Sharing among Intravenous Drug Abusers: National and International Perspectives*, National Institute on Drug Abuse Research Monograph 80, Washington, DC: Department of Health and Human Services Publication No. (ADM) 88–1567.

—— (1993) *The Indigenous Leader Outreach Model: Intervention Manual*, Washington, DC: National Institutes of Health Publication No. 93–3581.

Chapter 13

Peer-driven outreach to combat HIV among IDUs

A basic design and preliminary results

*Jean-Paul C. Grund, Robert S. Broadhead,
Douglas D. Heckathorn, L. Synn Stern
and Denise L. Anthony*

AIDS prevention efforts in the United States for out-of-treatment injection drug users (IDUs), other than a small number of activist-inspired needle exchanges, have relied almost entirely on a 'provider–client' model called 'street-based outreach'. The model consists of hiring a small number of community members, usually ex-users or people with street credentials, to contact and work with members of their own community as clients. They do this by going to neighbourhoods as 'outreach workers' (OWs) for the purpose of distributing prevention materials and information to IDUs, and recruiting them to various programmes and services, including research interviews conducted by social scientists.

In the first part of this chapter, we show that IDUs' responses to outreach efforts have been unexpectedly positive and have gone well beyond the expectations of being mere clients. Their responses indicate that future AIDS prevention efforts could well be based on a model that relies on an active collaboration with IDUs, and rewards them for working with their peers to reduce their risks of contracting and spreading HIV. We show that such a model would draw upon and strengthen the sharing rituals and norms of reciprocity that underlie and sustain user networks. Second, we describe the elements of such a prevention model, called a 'peer driven intervention' (PDI) (Broadhead and Heckathorn, 1994), which is based on the theory of 'group mediated social control' (Heckathorn, 1990). Third, we share some ethnographic data on the implementation and workings of a PDI recently started in the eastern United States. We conclude by discussing the potential of a PDI in addressing several other public health problems that involve 'hard to reach' populations who, like IDUs, could be expected to respond effectively to rewards for helping their peers help themselves.

AIDS PREVENTION AMONG IDUS

Research indicates that IDUs, on their own, began taking steps to protect themselves from the spread of HIV before governmentally sponsored outreach efforts began in the United States in 1988. For example, Des Jarlais *et al.* (1985) found in 1983 that IDUs in New York City began reacting to reports about the risk of AIDS by reducing needle sharing and increasing the demand for clean syringes. By 1984, IDUs' demand for clean needles was so great that it spawned a new market ripe for exploitation – needle sellers began re-packaging used needles and selling them as new (Des Jarlais *et al.*, 1985; Friedman *et al.*, 1987). In 1988, the federal government, through the National Institute on Drug Abuse (NIDA), began funding outreach projects in over sixty inner-city areas throughout the country, and substantial data documents that IDUs' response to them was impressive (Brown and Beschner, 1993). IDUs began to disinfect their needles with bleach and to reduce needle sharing. IDUs also increased their use of condoms, though less successfully. For example, in San Francisco during the winter/spring of 1986, *before* outreach distribution of bleach and condoms began, only 3 per cent of the city's estimated 15,000 IDUs reported that they regularly disinfected their syringes. OWs began distributing bleach in the streets in July, 1986. One year later, 55.4 per cent of IDUs interviewed reported using bleach and the percentage of IDUs not sharing needles increased from 9.8 per cent to 21 per cent (Watters *et al.*, 1990a). During that same year, only 4.3 per cent of the respondents reported using condoms at least half the time they had sex. By 1987, 32.7 per cent reported using condoms in general and 18.6 per cent reported using them at least half of the time. Watters *et al.* (1990b) reported that from the baseline measures taken in the winter/spring of 1986, there was a near doubling of HIV seroprevalence by early 1987, from 7 per cent to 13 per cent. After this point the curve is relatively flat through to late 1989. Watters *et al.* emphasised that 'major behaviour change occurred immediately following the implementation of outreach and bleach distribution' (Watters *et al.*, 1990b: 4).

Risk reduction by IDUs in response to outreach efforts in other cities was similarly significant, as researchers reported in New York City, Miami, Chicago, Denver, Baltimore, Cleveland, Hartford and other sites (NIDA, 1991; Brown and Beschner, 1993; Booth and Wiebel, 1992; Chitwood *et al.*, 1991; Neaigus *et al.*, 1990; Stephens *et al.*, 1991; Weeks *et al.*, 1990; Wiebel and Lampinen, 1991). Such changes occurred so rapidly following the implementation of outreach projects that secular trends, such as growing awareness of how HIV is transmitted, do not appear to be able to account for them. To control for the effects of secular trends, some studies used sequentially drawn samples, where one group (the quasi-control group) was interviewed for the pre-test at the same time that another group (the quasi-experimental group) was interviewed for the post-test. By comparing variations within the set of pre- and post-tests with variations across the pre- and post-tests, the design provided a control for secular trends such as general increases in the level of HIV prevention information. These studies offer further support for the conclusion that outreach helped to reduce high-risk drug-related behaviour. As Stephens *et al.* (1991: 570) reported in Cleveland:

For 19 of the 21 measures of risk associated with needle behaviour, the 'experimental' [post-test] group reported significantly lower levels of risk than the 'control' [contemporaneous pre-test] group. Similar contrasts were found in reduction of risk associated with general drug behaviours.

(See also Neaigus *et al.*, 1990)

Another study, by Booth and Wiebel (1992), provides further evidence of the independent impact of outreach projects. Outreach projects were implemented in Baltimore, Denver and El Paso beginning in 1987, all designed on the NADR Chicago model (see Chapter 12; Wiebel, 1988). Each project administered an initial and follow-up interview with samples of several hundred IDUs. However, in El Paso, due to 'agency problems' described by Broadhead and Heckathorn (1994), the outreach workers failed to access IDUs or even to sustain a presence in users' communities. Thus, in assessing the impact of outreach in the three cities, Booth and Wiebel (1992: 285) treated El Paso as a *de facto* control group in a quasi-experimental design, which led to the following conclusion:

That intervention through outreach could be effective was thus found not only in the significant risk reduction observed among subjects in Baltimore and Denver but in the relative lack of success in El Paso, which for the most part lacked the reinforcing presence of indigenous outreach staff.

In sum, research indicates that IDUs responded positively to outreach projects in making significant risk reduction changes, a response far greater than many experts ever expected. As Des Jarlais *et al.* (1991: 1279) concluded: 'Intravenous drug users have surprised many policy makers and researchers by exhibiting large-scale AIDS risk reduction.'

Indeed, IDUs' responsiveness went beyond risk reduction changes *per se*. In projects throughout the country, OWs found, and ethnographers documented, that IDUs volunteered and helped OWs carry out AIDS prevention efforts in many ways (Broadhead and Fox, 1990; Grund *et al.*, 1992; Rivera-Beckman, 1992; Johnson *et al.*, 1990). IDUs frequently introduced OWs to other users, and vouched for OWs in new communities. IDUs commonly helped OWs fill and prepare bleach bottles, and helped them distribute bleach, condoms and prevention information. It was also common for IDUs to aid OWs in locating users to be interviewed, or to find users who needed to return for follow-up interviews. As the directors of the San Francisco outreach project reported:

In short, the IV drug users became deeply involved in helping us gather health information regarding AIDS and its means of transmission. They generally looked favorably on such efforts to involve them voluntarily and encouraged their friends to cooperate in a similar fashion.

(Feldman and Biernacki, 1988: 31–32)

Similarly, in New York City, the Association for Drug Abuse Prevention and Treatment (ADAPT) reported that: 'users will often volunteer to help you set up your table and to bring their friends to it or distribute literature on the street' (ADAPT, n.d: 3). Ethnographers have even found operators of high-volume shooting galleries enforcing risk-reduction norms, as Ouellet *et al.* (1991: 80) described in Chicago:

Although Slim allows syringe sharing, he said, 'I discourage that', and he makes sure everyone who needs bleach has it ... To share a syringe in Slim's gallery is unusual; to share without first cleaning it with bleach violates gallery norms.

The Chicago outreach project concluded:

In fact, we have found that, as addicts become aware of the threat that AIDS poses, they are quite capable of assimilating a strong sense of social responsibility which can be readily channelled to include an assumed role of prevention advocacy.

(Wiebel, 1988: 147)

In sum, while outreach projects in many areas certainly promoted risk-reduction changes, IDUs and other drug-scene members clearly *augmented* those projects substantially. In the course of doing so, IDUs further disseminated and reinforced prevention norms within the larger IDU community.

The AIDS prevention efforts that IDUs engaged in on behalf of one another, and in helping OWs, can be seen as important extensions of various kinds of sharing patterns and norms of reciprocity that underlie and sustain user networks in the first place. One can describe the IDU subculture as a 'culture of survival', organised around the procurement of drugs (Grund, 1993). Due to their illicit and highly stigmatised status, drugs such as heroin and cocaine cannot be purchased in ordinary outlets. Drug users must turn to alternative sources – (often closed) illegal distribution networks which are at the bottom of the trafficking pyramid. Drugs are often sold by users to users, so the difference between the dealer and the client is ambiguous and protean. Drugs may also be sold by non-using street dealers. In both cases, retailers are necessarily highly distrustful of strangers or outsiders and they conceal their activities. Ritual interaction plays an important role in these networks to distinguish users from non-users and to prevent police detection (Carlson, 1977). As a result of entrepreneurial and law enforcement forces, these networks are generally unstable, both geographically and in time. Hence, the individual user needs up-to-date information on where the action is and the prevailing codes. This requires active and enduring participation in drug-use-defined networks. Active participation is further enhanced by a need to generate considerable amounts of money to pay black market drug prices, and to avoid the criminalisation and stigmatisation of injecting drug use.

While early descriptions of drug users conveyed a stereotypical predatory image, recent research shows that more prevalent interactional patterns evidence considerable cooperation and sharing (Grund, 1993). Habitual drug users are often organised in small, often dyadic friendship groups. These groups provide IDUs with opportunities for partnerships aimed at producing resources, through various hustles, to buy drugs. These friendship groups are linked to larger networks through exchanges and sharing of information, money, drugs and other necessities (Des Jarlais *et al.*, 1988; Preble and Casey, 1969). While the satisfaction of individual craving is an important objective of these interactions, they are also an expression of community solidarity, aimed at the maintenance of an interdependency network.

Needle sharing and its associated patterns of reciprocity provide a practical and emotional counter to the daily hardship of addict life (Grund, 1993; Grund *et al.*, 1991). Before AIDS, needle sharing fitted firmly into this pattern and was considered an expression of the almost universal subcultural code of '*share what you have*' (Wieder, 1974). Changing this hazardous practice has proven most successful when the changes do not contradict the subcultural norms. The introduction of bleach is a good example of an intervention that builds upon existing practice. It is even better when changes are initiated by group members themselves, as was witnessed at a Dutch needle exchange/outreach programme. After requests from participating IDUs, the programme started exchanging needles in bulk, allowing IDUs to share new needles with their peers and thereby conforming to the subcultural norm, yet in a safe way. Initial worries and objections from authorities and treatment facilities were found to be ungrounded. Monitoring of the programme found an exchange rate of 85 per cent and a very high retention rate: 52 per cent of bulk clients visited the programme twenty-five or more times. Ethnographic fieldwork established that the needles found their way to houses of IDUs who let friends and acquaintances get off. In addition to on-the-spot use, IDUs encouraged each other to take clean equipment home. Not infrequently, the provider of the needles was granted reciprocal gifts of drugs or other commodities (Grund *et al.*, 1992). The latter feature clearly demonstrates that this intervention was nested in prevalent patterns of sharing and reciprocity, characteristic of many interactions in IDU networks (Zule, 1992). Interventions that strengthen and build on patterns of IDUs' cooperation and reciprocity are likely to produce results beyond changing as individual IDU's risk behaviour.

Given IDUs' capabilities and responsiveness, new approaches to AIDS prevention that rely on, and work to strengthen, the capabilities of drug users to collaborate in promoting risk reduction among their peers are called for, as many AIDS researchers have been doing (Carlson and Needle, 1991; Chitwood *et al.*, 1991; Des Jarlais and Friedman, 1990; Feldman and Biernacki, 1988; Wiebel, 1988). Such prevention models would draw upon and strengthen the sharing rituals and reciprocity norms integral to user networks. For example, in the Netherlands several projects have involved former and active drug users and prostitutes working as peer educators (Trautmann, 1995). The Amsterdam-based user advocacy group, MDHG, recently received funding from the Dutch Ministry of Health to organise drug users into user groups aimed at changing subcultural health behaviour norms and advocating for users in general. In several German cities, chapters of JES (an advocacy group of 'users, ex-users and substituted [methadone] users') are running needle exchanges and low-threshold meeting centres (Hermann, 1993). In Australia, government-funded user groups in each state play a major role in the fight against AIDS (Herkt, 1993). Although anecdotal evidence and project-generated reports of the impact of these user groups is hopeful, systematic evaluations have not yet been undertaken.

While not totally absent in the United States, the involvement of user groups in promoting AIDS prevention and harm reduction practices has not significantly occurred, largely due to the severity of legal oppression of drug users (see Chapter-14). However, in contrast to traditional outreach and other projects based on a 'provider–client' model, a new approach, called a peer-driven intervention, has been developed and implemented in eastern Connecticut (Broadhead and Heckathorn, 1994). The model provides direct incentives to IDUs to invest effort in working with their peers to prevent AIDS, and also to perform many of the services that OWs do. The model represents, in the words of Rhodes (1993: 1319), a 'move from advocacy of health promotion towards an application of health promotion'. The theoretical underpinnings of this model are described below.

THE THEORY OF A PEER-DRIVEN INTERVENTION

The challenge posed by AIDS involves members of high-risk groups mobilising quickly for collective action to protect themselves. But collective action is a highly problematic achievement, especially for groups like IDUs who, due to the severity of legal oppression, have highly unstable memberships and great difficulty organising beyond that required in 'taking care of business' (Preble and Casey, 1969). At the beginning of the AIDS epidemic, the large size of the IDU populations in most cities, and their lack of organisation around public health issues, ensured that levels of collective action to combat AIDS would be low. In addition, several other factors were operating which made changing individuals' behaviour very difficult: the rewards of unsafe sex and getting high were powerful and immediate; the efficacy of safer practices in preventing HIV infection was uncertain; and the risk from any single act appeared to be small and long delayed (Lawlor, 1990). Furthermore, this new abstract hazard had to compete with a multitude of concrete problems typical of the IDU's daily life. Addressing HIV (e.g. by way of terminating needle sharing) flatly opposed well-established and functional community sharing norms dealing with risks that were far more apparent and immediately consequential, such as withdrawal or arrest on paraphernalia charges. These chronic threats scored significantly higher on IDUs' perceived hierarchy of risk than the remote and often poorly-understood risk of HIV infection. As Stern (1992: 124) has stated: 'with the constant threat of arrest, no housing and little income, AIDS just isn't the biggest problem on the block.' Even when HIV awareness and attempts at self-protection are manifest, these may be overruled by existing social norms of sharing (Barnard, 1993). Collective action among IDUs, therefore, tended to remain latent.

However, in light of the widely documented efforts IDUs *did* make to protect themselves, including their augmentation of outreach efforts, future AIDS prevention efforts would be strengthened significantly if means were found to catalyse or facilitate the process by which IDUs mobilise for collective action. Such means would speed the process by which a latent group, like IDUs, are able to identify common interests and create and enforce AIDS prevention norms consistent with community codes.

A new development in the theory of collective action, the *theory of group-mediated social control* (Heckathorn, 1988, 1990), shows how this might be achieved. According to this theory, relationships of power are never strictly dyadic. Virtually all individuals are members of groups with whom they are interdependent. These include groups of family members, friends, neighbours, co-workers and others with whom individuals interact regularly. To the extent that members of a group are interdependent, sanctions or other means of control directed at any individual have consequences that extend to other group members. For example, when one person is promoted in a job or fired, the sanction spills over and affects family members and friends. Except in the limited case of social isolates, almost all social sanctions targeted at an actor generate collective rewards or punishments that impinge on his or her primary group. Imprisonment is an example of a punishment that spills over to others. It is not merely a personal calamity; it frequently drives the families of inmates into poverty. Similarly, rewards spill over to peers. When a family's major breadwinner earns an important promotion, the life chances of all family members may improve. Due to the spillover of rewards and punishments from targeted individuals to their significant peers, social sanctions are not individualised at all. Instead, they give rise to collective rewards or collective punishments.

Given that most social sanctioning includes both an individual and a collective component, behavioural compliance can arise from either of two theoretically distinguishable sources (see Figure 13.1). First, it can arise from individual-sanction-based control that is exercised by an agent such as a teacher, police officer, parent or neighbour and directed at the actor who is the target of control. For example, the agent may threaten the targeted actor with punishment or offer the promise of reward. The result is a dyadic power relation of the sort presumed in many sociological analyses of power

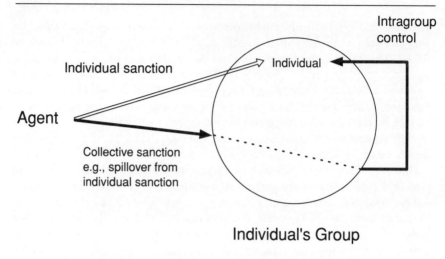

Figure 13.1 Individual versus group-mediated social control

relations. Second, compliance can also arise from group-mediated control (Heckathorn, 1990), as when students obey teachers because punishment administered by the school would be augmented by parents; or when workers hold onto disagreeable jobs because unemployment would inflict hardship on their families. In these cases, the agent of authority's influence is amplified by the group in which the target of control is embedded.

The traditional emphasis on individual incentives in studies of social and organisational control is overdrawn (Heckathorn, 1990). Individual incentives alone do not suffice to ensure compliance in complex organisations or communities. Large-scale compliance is much more likely when official sanctions are reinforced by internal selective incentive systems. Hence, group-mediated social control is a prerequisite for effective legal, organisational, or normative control. Control based on individual sanctions works by altering people's *inclinations*, that is, their preferences regarding their own personal behaviour. It does this by using what may be termed *primary incentives*, such as performance-specific rewards or punishments. In contrast, group-mediated social control works by altering people's *regulatory interests*, that is, their preferences regarding how others should behave. Group-mediated control does this by using what may be termed *secondary incentives*, such as rewards or punishments based on the performance of peers.

Collective action of a group can be promoted by using secondary incentives to amplify the regulatory interests that group members may share but are not acting on. If that amplification is sufficient in magnitude, what had been a latent group will begin to act collectively. For example, a latent group at risk of contracting HIV may become capable of creating and enforcing further norms with which to control high-risk behaviour. Below, we describe how this can be done in practice.

PRELIMINARY RESULTS OF A PEER-DRIVEN INTERVENTION (PDI)

A PDI to combat HIV has begun in eastern Connecticut (Broadhead and Heckathorn, 1994). It is designed to reward IDUs for performing the essential functions of OWs, using a combination of primary and secondary incentives. The incentives are also meant to promote self-organisation among IDUs by enhancing positive forms of interaction within their own community.

The first task of traditional outreach is recruiting IDUs into prevention programmes, where the nexus of the PDI is a storefront that provides HIV testing and counselling, harm reduction education, and prevention materials. In the PDI, IDUs are motivated to recruit other users for the above services via a coupon system: for each IDU recruited bearing a coupon, the user who *recruited* the person receives a modest monetary reward. Only modest rewards are required, because the costs involved in exercising influence over peers is usually small, and there now exists widespread concern about AIDS and its threat to the welfare of peers.

Each recruit, in turn, is also given a limited number of coupons to recruit more IDUs within their network. Thus, the mechanism co-opts user networks to serve as a medium to recruit further IDUs. If adequate incentives are employed – we are giving each user three coupons worth $10 per referral – the expanding system of chain-referrals may be robust enough to saturate the IDU population. In addition, all members of the IDU community are given an equal opportunity to participate in the intervention and be rewarded for doing so.

The peer-recruitment mechanism has several advantages over relying on paid staffs of OWs. First, it puts the burden of identifying recruits on those with the best current information: active users. Of course, users vary in their centrality in the IDU community, so they can be expected to vary in the success of their recruitment efforts. However, the combined efforts of multiple users provides for an exponential exploration of potential recruits, while the one-to-one worker–client basis, typical of outreach, 'allows only [for] arithmetic progression into the target population, limiting the numbers who can be effectively reached' (Stimson *et al.*, 1994).

Second, the pay-for-performance design of the PDI rewards the most productive recruiters, and recruiters are paid in direct proportion to the success of their efforts. Those who recruit no one receive nothing.

Third, with IDUs accessing their peers, the PDI recruitment effort is always couched in terms that are culturally appropriate to each user subgroup.

Another central task of traditional outreach projects is distributing AIDS prevention information. Outreach programmes educate IDUs both in the field and through education modules on HIV, STDs, the proper use of bleach, and so on, at a storefront, van, or similar space. In the PDI, IDUs are given incentives to educate their peers in the community. When recruits come to the storefront, the programme staff administers a short knowledge test to measure the extent to which recruits passed on specific information they were given about AIDS and the PDI to their recruits. Recruiters can earn up to $10 for a recruit who scores well on the knowledge test. Thus, for both recruiting and educating three peers, a recruiter can earn up to $60. Highly successful peer recruiters/educators (with emphasis on the latter function) are offered another set of coupons.

Rewarding recruiters for educating peers in the community has several advantages over the efforts of staffs of OWs. First, it puts the responsibility for educating IDUs on those who are most likely to be influential: their peers. Second, one of the most effective ways of motivating students to invest in a body of knowledge is to have them teach one another (Juzang, 1992). Third, peers educating peers entails considerable repetition. Subjects are first educated by their peer-recruiter, then by project staff, and subsequently subjects rehearse what they have learned when educating and recruiting their peers. Finally, when recruiters come in to collect their earned reward, they are given a second knowledge test and possible misunderstandings and gaps in knowledge are corrected.

A final task of outreach is distributing AIDS prevention materials such as bleach and condoms. In the PDI, each IDU following their education is offered large quantities of prevention materials, asked to give them to their peers and encouraged to return for more. Thus, the PDI is able to flood a user population quickly and continuously with prevention supplies.

Preliminary ethnographic results of the first two operating months of the PDI are encouraging. As a result of negative local press coverage, very little energy was necessary to establish the initial pool of respondents/peer recruiters – these first subjects were attracted by the stories about the project in the newspaper, and they started checking out the storefront even before it opened. Some people left a note under the storefront door, showing their eagerness to meet with the project, such as the following: 'We come by at 1.41. You never open. We're junkies – no patients. Comprendo.' Although the project is the first in its kind anywhere, and almost all of the first fifty respondents interviewed stated they had never been interviewed before on matters regarding drug use or sexuality, the level of distrust seems fairly low. Only a few potential respondents exhibited reservations or had questions about confidentiality, which were easily satisfied. However, as was anticipated, some anxiety about contact with the project exists in the community; some respondents/peer recruiters explained that some of their friends do not trust the project and expressed fears of being reported violating parole, as one explained:

They think you are police and have cameras in the office ... The other day two of you walked down the street and one guy said 'They are narcs, yes, even her' ... Nah, there are no cameras in here, that was paranoid shit.

Although the interview and education session requires a considerable investment of time by each respondent – the whole session takes about two to two-and-a-half hours – no one has walked out of the session and almost everyone seems to appreciate the opportunity for reflection. Respondents say they like the interview. As one user noted: 'It really covers all important things.' Many have said that they learned something new and readily useful from the education component, as explained by another respondent:

I'll be honest with you. I came in because of the money, and also because you seemed nice people. I was curious about the whole thing. But I'm really glad I came in, because I really learned some things I did not know before. And it made me start thinking about things, sitting down and talking about everything. You don't do that normally when you are out there, you get sort of desensitised.

Getting respondents into treatment is not a priority of the programme. However, at least two respondents – one on her way to an intake, and another who phoned after his admission – claimed that going through the education and interview session made them decide to enter treatment.

Although, as indicated by the previous quote, the financial compensation is an important incentive to come in for an interview, many respondents are eager to participate in the recruitment and education of their peers. They are aware of their superior ability to reach other IDUs (as compared to professional outreach) and feel they can play an important role in preventing HIV infection. As one female respondent explained: 'Maybe that's one thing I can do. Stopping some people getting infected.'

Finally, the project reaches a group of people who may be at risk of HIV but do not fall within the study criteria. For example, a growing number of teens and young adults find their way to the storefront to pick up free condoms, discuss sex and ask questions about HIV.

CONCLUSION

We have outlined above an alternative to traditional AIDS outreach based on a form of secondary-incentive-based organisation termed a 'peer-driven intervention'. Of course, a definitive assessment of the strengths and weaknesses of the PDI must await more extensive empirical results. Should the results prove positive, similar interventions might be devised to address other public health problems. A PDI appears most promising when clear performance measures are available, and *any* of the following three conditions are met:

1 It is extremely difficult, time consuming, and costly for outreach workers or ethnographers to tap into innumerable local networks. Knowledge is usually highly localised when activities are intimate, normatively suspect and controversial;

2 Individuals lack strong conventional ties, and rely instead on peer support. For example, the unemployed cannot be reached in the workplace, and drop-outs cannot be reached in schools. Yet unless they are social isolates, they can be reached through peers;

3 Individual behaviour is subject to peer control. Few individuals will change their behaviour at the cost of ridicule from peers, but this problem does not arise when the change is initiated through peers.

A major area of potential application of secondary-incentive-based organisation is the delivery of human services. For example, PDIs like the one described above may be appropriate in combating an array of public health problems in the community, including accessing pregnant teenagers in need of prenatal care, parents whose children have not been immunised, or runaway/homeless youths. It can also be adapted to broad-based hypertension screening, in an intervention in which chronic patients provide preventive care for their peers. The prerequisite is that individuals must have information on, and influence over, others who live with the same problem. As conventionally viewed, out-of-treatment IDUs might seem to be the least promising candidates for assistance based on self-help. Yet their response in helping one another protect themselves from HIV suggests that such approaches should be explored much more extensively. If IDUs can help themselves, other groups can do so as well.

REFERENCES

ADAPT (Association for Drug Abuse Prevention and Treatment) (n.d.) 'Street outreach tactics: the do's and dont's', New York City, unpublished paper.

Barnard, M. A. (1993) 'Needle sharing in context: patterns of sharing among men and women injectors and HIV risks', *Addiction*, 88: 805–812.

Booth, R. and Wiebel, W. (1992) 'Effectiveness of reducing needle-related risks for HIV through indigenous outreach to injection drug users', *American Journal on Addictions*, 1: 277–287.

Broadhead, R. S. and Fox, K. J. (1990) 'Takin' it to the streets: AIDS outreach as ethnography', *Journal of Contemporary Ethnography*, 19: 322–348.

Broadhead, R. S. and Heckathorn, D. D. (1994) 'AIDS prevention outreach among injection drug users: agency problems and new approaches', *Social Problems*, 41: 3.

Brown, B. and Beschner, G. M. (1993) *Handbook on Risk of AIDS: Injection Drug Users and Sexual Partners*, Westport, CT: Greenwood Press.

Carlson, K. A. (1977) 'Identifying the stranger: An analysis of behavioural rules for sales of heroin', in B.M. Du Toit (ed.) *Drugs, Rituals and Altered States of Consciousness*, Rotterdam: Balkema.

Carlson, G. and Needle, R. (1991) 'Sponsoring addict self-organization (Addicts

Against AIDS): A case study', in *Community-Based AIDS Prevention: Studies of Intravenous Drug Users and Their Sexual Partners: Proceedings of the First Annual NADR National Meeting*, Washington, DC: National Institute on Drug Abuse, US Government Printing Office (DHHS Pub. no. 80M–91–1752).

Chitwood, D. D., Comerford, M., Khoury, E. L. and Vogel, J. A. (1991) 'Behaviour changes of intravenous drug users after an intervention program', in *Community-Based AIDS Prevention: Studies of Intravenous Drug Users and Their Sexual Partners: Proceedings of the First Annual NADR National Meeting*, Washington, DC: National Institute on Drug Abuse, US Government Printing Office (DHHS Pub. no. 80M–91–1752).

Des Jarlais, D. C. and Friedman, S. R. (1990) 'Shooting galleries and AIDS: Infection probabilities and "tough" policies', *American Journal of Public Health*, 80: 142–145.

Des Jarlais, D. C., Friedman, S. R. and Hopkins, W. (1985) 'Risk reduction for AIDS among intravenous drug users', *Annals of Internal Medicine*, 103: 755–759.

Des Jarlais, D. C., Friedman, S. R., Sotheran, J. L. and Stoneburger, R. (1988) 'The sharing of drug injection equipment and the AIDS epidemic in New York City: The first decade', in R. J. Battjes and R. W. Pickins (eds) *Needle Sharing among Intravenous Drug Abusers: National and International Perspectives*, Rockville, MD: NIDA.

Des Jarlais, D. C., Abdul-Quader, A. and Tross, S. (1991) 'The next problem: Maintenance of AIDS risk reduction among intravenous drug users', *International Journal of the Addictions*, 26: 1279–1292.

Feldman, H. W. and Biernacki, P. (1988) 'The ethnography of needle sharing among intravenous drug users and implications for public policies and intervention strategies', in R. J. Battjes and R. W. Pickens (eds) *Needle Sharing among Intravenous Drug Abusers: National and International Perspectives, National Institute on Drug Abuse Research Monograph No. 80*, Washington, DC: US Government Printing Office.

Friedman, S. R., Des Jarlais, D. C., Sotheran, J. C., Garber, J., Cohen, H. and Smith, D. (1987) 'AIDS and self-organization among intravenous drug users', *International Journal of the Addictions*, 22: 201–219.

Grund, J-P. C. (1993) *Drug Use as a Social Ritual: Functionality, Symbolism and Determinants of Self-Regulation*, Rotterdam: Instituut voor Verslavingsonderzoek (IVO).

Grund, J-P. C., Kaplan, C. D., Adriaans, N. F. P. and Blanken, P. (1991) 'Drug sharing and HIV transmission risks: The practice of "frontloading" in the Dutch injecting drug user population', *Journal of Psychoactive Drugs*, 23: 1–10.

Grund, J-P. C., Blanken, P., Adriaans, N. F. P., Kaplan, C. D., Barendregt, C. and Meeuwsen, M. (1992) 'Reaching the unreached: Targeting hidden IDU populations with clean needles via known users', *Journal of Psychoactive Drugs*, 24(1): 41–47.

—— (1988) 'Collective sanctions and the emergence of prisoner's dilemma norms', *American Journal of Sociology*, 94: 535–562.

Heckathorn, D. D. (1990) 'Collective sanctions and compliance norms: A formal theory of group-mediated social control', *American Sociological Review*, 55: 366–384.

Herkt, D. (1993) 'Peer-based user groups: The Australian experience', in N. Heather, A. Wodak, E. Nadelmann and P. O'Hare (eds) *Psychoactive Drugs & Harm Reduction: From Faith to Science*, London: Whurr Publishers.

Hermann, W. (1993) 'The working of J.E.S. (Junkies, Ex-junkies, Substituted), structure, scope and aims of the network', paper presented at IV International Conference on the Reduction of Drug Related Harm, Rotterdam.

Johnson, J., Williams, M. L. and Kotarba, J. A. (1990) 'Proactive and reactive strategies for delivering community-based HIV prevention services: An ethnographic analysis', *AIDS Education and Prevention*, 2: 191–200.

Juzang, I. (1992) 'Reaching the hip-hop generation', unpublished manuscript, MEE Productions, Philadelphia.

Lawlor, E. J. (1990) 'When a possible job becomes impossible: Politics, public health, and the management of the AIDS epidemic', in E. C. Hargrove and J. C. Glidewell (eds) *Impossible Jobs in Public Management*, Kansas City, MD: University Press of Kansas.

Neaigus, A., Sufian, M., Friedman, S. R., Goldsmith, D. S., Stepherson, B., Mota, P., Pascal, J. and Des Jarlais, D. C. (1990) 'Effects of outreach intervention on risk reduction among intravenous drug users', *AIDS Education and Prevention*, 2: 253–271.

NIDA (National Institute on Drug Abuse) (1991) 'NIDA's AIDS projects succeed in reaching drug addicts, changing high-risk behaviours', *NIDA NOTES*, 6: 25–27.

Ouellet, L. J., Jimenez, A. D., Johnson, W. A. and Wiebel, W. W. (1991) 'Shooting galleries and HIV disease: Variations in places for injecting illicit drugs', *Crime and Delinquency*, 37: 64–85.

Preble, E. D. and Casey, J. H. (1969) 'Taking care of business – The heroin user's life on the streets', *International Journal of the Addictions*, 4(1): 11–24.

Rhodes, T. (1993) 'Time for community change: What has outreach to offer?', *Addiction*, 88: 1317–1320.

Rivera-Beckman, J. (1992) 'Community outreach in the time of AIDS: The San Francisco, Chicago and POCAAN models: A report to the New York State Division of substance abuse services', unpublished manuscript, National Development Research Institute, New York City.

Stephens, R. C., Feucht, T. E. and Roman, S. W. (1991) 'Effects of an intervention program on AIDS-related drug and needle behavior among intravenous drug users', *American Journal of Public Health*, 81: 568–571.

Stern, L. S. (1992) 'Self-injection education for street-level sex workers', in P. O'Hare, R. Newcombe, E. Buning, E. Drucker and A. Matthews (eds) *Reducing the Harm from Drug Use*, London: Routledge.

Stimson, G. V., Eaton, G., Rhodes, T. J. and Power, R. (1994) 'Potential development of community oriented HIV outreach among drug injectors in the UK', *Addiction*, 89: 1601–1611.

Trautmann, F. (1995) 'Peer support as a method of risk reduction in injecting drug user communities', *Journal of Drug Issues*, 25: 617–28.

Watters, J. K., Downing, M., Case, P., Lorvick, J., Cheng Y-T. and Fergusson, B. (1990a) 'AIDS prevention for intravenous drug users in the community: Street-based education and risk behaviour', *American Journal of Community Psychology*, 18: 587–596.

Watters, J. K., Cheng, Y-T., Segal, M., Lorvick, J., Case, P., Taylor, F. and Carlson, J. R. (1990b) 'Epidemiology and prevention of HIV in heterosexual IV drug users in San Francisco, 1986–1989', paper presented at VIth International Conference on AIDS, San Francisco.

Weeks, M. R., Singer, M., Schensul, J. J., Jia, Z. and Grier, M. (1990) 'Project COPE: Preventing AIDS among injection drug users and their sexual partners: Comprehensive data report', unpublished manuscript, Project COPE, Hartford, CT.

Wiebel, W. W. (1988) 'Combining ethnographic and epidemiologic methods in targeted AIDS interventions: The Chicago model', in R. J. Battjes and R. W. Pickens (eds) *Needle Sharing among Intravenous Drug Abusers: National and International Perspectives, National Institute on Drug Abuse Research Monograph No. 80*, Washington, DC.: US Government Printing Office.

Wiebel, W. W. and Lampinen, T. M. (1991) 'Primary prevention of HIV/1 among intravenous drug users', *Journal of Primary Prevention*, 12: 35–48.
Wieder D. L. (1974) 'Telling the code', in R. Turner (ed.) *Ethnomethodology: Selected Readings*, Harmondsworth: Penguin Education.
Zule, W. A. (1992) 'Risk and reciprocity: HIV and the injection drug user', *Journal of Psychoactive Drugs*, 24(3): 243–249.

Chapter 14

Collective organisation of injecting drug users and the struggle against AIDS

Benny Jose, Samuel R. Friedman, Alan Neaigus, Richard Curtis, Meryl Sufian, Bruce Stepherson and Don C. Des Jarlais

Injecting drug users (IDUs) become infected with HIV in a limited number of ways: by sharing syringes or other paraphernalia in direct interactions with others; by injecting drugs with contaminated injection equipment previously used by unknown IDUs at shooting galleries, dealer houses, abandoned buildings, or at outside locations (Marmor *et al.*, 1987; Schoenbaum *et al.*, 1989); by having the drug mixture for two or more IDUs prepared for injection in a previously used syringe (Jose *et al.*, 1993); or by unprotected sex. In all of these patterns except when sharing contaminated equipment used by unknown IDUs, risk behaviour involves direct social interaction between two or more individuals and therefore allows for social pressure to come into play. Even in situations where direct social interaction between IDUs does not occur, the sharing of injection equipment is influenced by the dynamics of core institutions of the drug subculture such as various indoor or outdoor gathering places where drugs and equipment are bought and/or used by a number of IDUs (perhaps from different friendship groups). Normative and other pressures also occur in these settings. Ethnographic studies have provided a detailed picture of the complexity of these interactions (McKeganey and Barnard, 1992; Grund, 1993).

A wide range of intervention strategies which focus on the individual have been initiated by public health agencies and other non-user organisations among IDUs. These methods include street outreach (Neaigus *et al.*, 1990a; Abdul-Quader *et al.*, 1992), treatment oriented approaches, and syringe exchange (Dolan *et al.*, 1993; Des Jarlais and Friedman, 1992b; Hartgers *et al.*, 1989). In many places, IDUs have reduced their risk of acquiring or transmitting HIV by adopting safer injection techniques (Becker and Joseph, 1988; CDC, 1991; Des Jarlais and Friedman, 1992a) and safe sex practices. Sexual behaviour changes such as always using condoms, however, have lagged behind safer injection practices (Jain *et al.*, 1989; Sibthorpe, 1992; Watkins *et al.*, 1993). This has been the case in most locations irrespective of the history of the epidemic, seroprevalence or type of intervention strategy adopted (Des Jarlais *et al.*, 1992). Even among IDUs who have reduced risk, risk-free behaviours have been difficult to maintain over a long time (Des Jarlais, *et al.*, 1991) and 'relapse' into risk behaviour was not unusual. These point to the limitations of intervention models which focus exclusively on the individual, and the need for interventions to look beyond the individual, to focus on the social contexts of risk behaviours.

A broad range of factors can influence risk behaviour among IDUs at different levels. At the interpersonal level, type and intimacy of relationship between IDUs have been found to be important. For example, consistent condom use has been particularly hard to implement among IDUs, especially in intimate regular partnerships as opposed to more casual or commercial sexual encounters (Sibthorpe, 1992; Watkins *et al.*, 1993). In our recent research on consistent condom use in sexual relationships of IDUs, we found that condoms were used less consistently in 'very close' relationships (Friedman *et al.*, 1993b).

Risk behaviours are also influenced by social, structural, and situational factors such as the institutional and market needs of shooting galleries and drug dealers; the relationships between drug injectors and their families and neighbours; the extent to which society has stigmatised drug use so that drug injecting is carried out furtively and quickly rather than more carefully; police pressures; and the extent to which drug injectors have jobs, other legal income and housing. In Madrid and New York City, for example, IDUs who lack legal income are more likely to inject with syringes others have used (Friedman *et al.*, 1993c), and in New York condom use is lower among homeless drug injectors (Friedman *et al.*, 1993b).

Research shows that risk behaviours and risk reduction are social acts that are influenced by one's peers. Friedman *et al.* (1987) first provided evidence that deliberate risk reduction by IDUs was more likely among those whose peers were also reducing their drug injection risk. Abdul-Quader *et al.* (1990) and Tross *et al.* (1992) have shown similar results for deliberate sexual risk reduction among IDUs and their sexual partners. Others have shown that HIV risk behaviours are influenced by the attitudes and behaviours of peers (Neaigus *et al.*, 1990b; Sotheran, 1991). The probability that IDUs will share syringes, for example, is greater if they have a closer social relationship and/or if they have known each other for a long time, and the norms of IDU peer groups can encourage syringe sharing (as in dictating that they rotate who first uses a syringe) as well as discourage it (as in holding that true friends do not share syringes with each other, Neaigus *et al.*, 1993). Consistent condom use has also been found to be higher in relationships where IDUs report that their peer culture did not discourage it (Friedman *et al.*, 1993b).

Taken as a whole, this suggests that risk reduction is a product not simply of individual behaviour but of social norms and peer culture as well. Thus, we need to devise ways to influence peer culture.

MODELS OF SOCIAL INTERVENTION

Friedman *et al.* (1994) have argued that cultures of risk can be changed by several social processes. These include social diffusion; opinion-leader-focused outreach, in which pre-existing subcultural and peer leaders are recruited to promulgate risk reduction and norms; collective self-organisation to change risk cultures, as can be produced by social movements (e.g. drug users' organisations); and changes in the wider social environment. Here we will briefly discuss the first two of these – diffusion and leadership-focused outreach – before considering attempts to organise drug users to mobilise against AIDS and to change their social situations.

Diffusion theory

Diffusion has been a widely discussed model of cultural change in anthropology and sociology (Ogburn, 1922; Rogers, 1982; Rogers and Shoemaker, 1971). Diffusion theory points to several issues as salient for public health interventions in a subculture. It is necessary first to understand the subculture well enough to predict or devise innovations that will be acceptable. Second, it is necessary to develop ways to monitor how the subculture both uses innovations and changes itself as a result; and finally, it is important to introduce alterations in the innovation or in the way in which it is presented if the monitoring uncovers problems.

The San Francisco model of HIV-focused outreach to drug injectors is an example of a diffusion-based HIV intervention (Newmeyer *et al.*, 1989; Broadhead and Fox, 1990). Based on earlier research among San Francisco drug users, it was decided that the use of bleach as a decontaminant of syringes would be accepted by the user subculture (Newmeyer, 1988). To spread this innovation, the project staff first used word-of-mouth education, assuming that this would lead to widespread bleach use. They soon realised, however, that outreach workers would have to distribute bleach to get the innovation accepted and disseminated (Newmeyer *et al.*, 1989). While spreading this norm, project staff took extra care that there should be minimal disruption of the established norms, values and procedures of drug injection among IDUs (Broadhead, 1991).

This project may have been successful in slowing the spread of HIV among San Francisco IDUs. Bleach use became quite widespread among IDUs in this city, although many drug injectors responded to the project by reducing the extent to which they injected with syringes that others had used. While seroprevalence had been rising prior to the introduction of this innovation, it subsequently levelled off at about 12 per cent (Watters *et al.*, 1990).

Leadership-focused models

Leadership-focused models aim to encourage pre-existing group leaders to champion an innovation by recruiting influential persons to advocate health-oriented behaviours (see Chapter 11). The behaviours to be advocated have to be acceptable to the subculture (as in diffusion models), but considerable emphasis is placed on how local leaders will react to the innovations. Ways have to be found to get local leaders to spend time and perhaps to risk their credibility on behalf of the innovation. The problems that leaders face in advocating an innovation – such as whether it falls outside the domain of their normal patterns of personal interaction – thus become questions that can help focus the practical discussions and problem-solving efforts of public health theorists and practitioners.

Local leadership has to be identified in order to recruit individuals to take part. For interventions among gay men and drug users such projects usually should not focus on the formal leaders of a community (Morales and Fullilove, 1992). Indeed, formal leaders may have to be circumvented or even openly opposed, since many are removed from the daily lives of those in the surrounding community (Quimby and Friedman, 1989). It is usually a question of recruiting the opinion leaders on a given city block, within a given friendship group, or a particular network of drug injectors. A detailed understanding of local social relationships may be needed to identify such leaders. This may require a substantial effort in direct observation of, and intimate association with, the target group. Ethnographic and sociometric techniques may help in both identifying and recruiting the persons who are able to persuade others to accept risk-reducing innovations.

Once selected, local leaders need training about substantive health issues so that they can answer questions and disarm opposition. Advocating change may endanger their prestige and standing, so they need to agree with the importance of the health issue and the efficacy of the intervention and develop ways to maintain or increase their own standing by advocating 'necessary' changes. Often, the local leaders will find ways to improve upon any model which health professionals have devised. On other occasions, however, the needs of local leaders might alter the behavioural changes that are recommended in harmful ways. If a large proportion of local leaders are unable or unwilling to work effectively towards risk reduction, then other techniques might be more appropriate.

Leadership-focused models have been applied in a number of areas of health intervention, including interventions around coronary health in North Karelia, Finland (McAlister et al., 1982; Puska et al., 1985); AIDS interventions among IDUs (see Chapter 11; Wiebel, 1988; Wiebel et al., 1989); and AIDS interventions among gay men (See Chapter 6; Kelly et al., 1991, 1992). These leadership-focused intervention models have been found to be effective in bringing about health-related behavioural changes among participants.

Leadership-focused interventions, however, may face certain practical problems in their implementation. If hierarchies of influence change rapidly, or if social networks are short-lived (such that social relationships are transient), or if there is serious resistance to change among influential segments of a subculture, leadership-focused approaches may have less of a behavioural impact. Social movements or projects aimed at changing the larger social environment might then be more effective.

Collective organising for normative and behavioural change

Communities often respond to threats by organising a group response. When the threat is observably from other human beings or from dominant social institutions, these organisations take the form of pressure groups, social movements or collective action projects (Tilly, 1978).

Gay men and lesbians were the first groups to set up intensive self-help organisations to fight against AIDS. Since gays had formed organisations (such as gay networks, retail establishments, newspapers and other institutions) in the 1970s as part of this response, by the time HIV became a visible threat to their community in the 1980s, they had a pre-existing foundation of organisational strength to respond to the epidemic (Adam, 1987; Kayal, 1993). Gay organisations throughout the world have been instrumental not only in making their members aware of the risk of HIV during the early stages of the epidemic, but also in speaking for the interests of the gay community and generating governmental and policy responses. As a result, gays in many cities with affiliational ties to these organisations have considerably reduced their risk of contracting the virus (Altman, 1991; Coutinho et al., 1989; Stall et al., 1988).

Drug injectors have had a very different organisational infrastructure from gay men. Their primary organisational forms have been those of the underground drug market itself – dealers' networks, shooting galleries and the like – which have provided neither the economic resources nor the 'safe space' for communal organising activities. Prior to the AIDS epidemic, there were sizeable drug users' organisations only in the Netherlands. In spite of the hostility faced by drug injectors and their lack of resources, drug users' organisations have emerged as important players in the fight against AIDS.

The history of efforts to change IDUs' culture of risk by establishing drug users' organisations to mobilise for subcultural change suggests that there have been two distinct patterns of development. In one, drug users organise on their own, perhaps with encouragement or financial support from official sources. In the other, interventions are organised by outsiders to assist IDUs who are not otherwise setting up drug users' organisations. The remainder of this chapter will briefly review the history of autonomous self-organisation efforts by drug users around the world; discuss a case study of an effort to organise IDUs from the outside in Brooklyn, New York, and present data from an outcome evaluation of its behavioural impact (with particular focus on changes in condom use); and consider what remains to be learned about drug users organising against HIV.

AUTONOMOUS DRUG USERS' ORGANISATIONS

The earliest drug users' organisations were formed in the Netherlands in the 1970s, and there were approximately thirty to forty active users' groups in Dutch cities when AIDS first became a visible concern in 1983–84 (Friedman *et al.*, 1993a). Currently, the countries with the strongest drug users' organisations are probably Germany and Australia, although there are also groups in the United Kingdom, the Netherlands, Denmark, Norway, France, Belgium, Italy, Spain, Slovenia, Switzerland, Hungary, Lithuania, New Zealand and the United States. Efforts are also under way to organise groups in several developing countries.

The European users' groups have organised a coalition, the European Interest Group of Drug Users, while a worldwide federation – the International Drug Users Network – was formed in 1992. These federations attempt to work towards increasing recognition of IDUs' basic human rights, to keep the various drug users' groups aware of each other's activities, to encourage the growth of new groups, to represent users' views at public forums, and to influence public and private policies that affect drug users.

Activities

Drug users' organisations have engaged in a number of activities, which have often explicitly been aimed at changing users' norms, beliefs and practices in ways that can retard or prevent HIV spread. Most groups have engaged in extensive outreach activities in which they have conducted street education and distributed risk reduction supplies such as syringes and condoms. Indeed, they are often major participants in local syringe exchange efforts. Many of these groups use newsletters as a strategy of education and as a way to organise their activities and to attract support, while some have made similar use of videos (Burrows and Price, 1993; Friedman, 1993). Users' groups have also been involved in helping develop national and local programmes of HIV prevention and of caring for those affected by HIV. In Baltimore, for example, a users' group has used a street newsletter as a major focus of activities, but has also been involved in running a home for homeless users and has taken part in demonstrations associated with social welfare issues affecting drug users.

Context

In some countries, such as the Netherlands, drug users' organisations have arisen autonomously. In others, such as in Australia, they have arisen semi-spontaneously where drug users take the initiative to start a group and quickly receive sponsorship or funding from public health agencies. In many cities or countries, drug users' organisations have not arisen at all. While the processes which affect the probability that users will organise have not been widely studied, the work of Burrows and Price (1993) and of Friedman *et al.* (1988) suggest that a variety of factors are of particular importance in affecting whether drug users' organisations arise and how successful they become. These include the general social climate, and whether it encourages hostility to, stigmatisation of and self-blame among drug users. Where drug users are widely viewed as despicable, public hostility makes it more difficult for them to organise openly and makes it less likely that their efforts will lead to the visible successes that are invaluable in sustaining morale and enthusiasm for any organising effort. Intervention factors also include level of police repression of drug users' activities, the extent to which users have access to food, shelter and other resources through social welfare systems or employment, the extent to which users have access to methadone and other substitution therapy, and the extent to which public health, church or political organisations provide resources.

Organising capability is thus in part determined by whether users have the time, money and operational freedom to take part in organisational activities. Organising requires time to talk with other members of the group about organisational issues, a location in which to hold both small and large meetings, and money and equipment to write and produce newsletters. Where police pressure, for example, deprives users of time and money, organising becomes problematic. In contrast, where substitution therapy (e.g. methadone maintenance) provides more time and a greater likelihood of employment, and where public health agencies provide resources, organising is facilitated.

The size of the local user community and the organisational experience of its members also can affect organising success. In many large cities, there are sufficient drug injectors for there to be a considerable pool of talent available, if it can be mobilised. In smaller cities or towns there is usually a smaller pool of experienced leaders, but the correspondingly smaller size of the drug user community may make it easier to establish ties with most other users and thus to develop effective action. Many of the European and Australian users' groups are in small cities. In the United States, many drug injectors have political or organisational experience from the 1960s (as members, for example, of the Black Panthers or other radical groups), or from religious groups (such as the Nation of Islam), or from neighbourhood organisations. The initial organisers of the Dutch *junkiebonden* had experience based in radical youth groups. This provides an initial basis for effective leadership. To the extent to which this leadership is able to maintain or establish wide social networks, and to find issues or projects around which to mobilise other users, it can involve large numbers of drug users in its activities, including those which aim at risk-reducing subcultural change (Friedman, 1993).

There have to date been no formal studies of the impact of drug users' organisations on risk behaviours of local drug-injecting communities and networks, or on how the different strategic choices made by these organisations might affect the extent of risk reduction among IDUs. Clearly, such research would be valuable, but it is difficult to organise and conduct, and it is also often difficult to fund. This is nonetheless an important area for future research.

ORGANISING IDUs FROM THE OUTSIDE: A CASE STUDY

This section briefly describes an effort at 'outside organising' among IDUs in New York City. The Community AIDS Prevention Outreach Demonstration (CAPOD) project, which initiated the organising efforts, was one of the New York components of the National AIDS Demonstration Research (NADR) programme. CAPOD was implemented by National Development and Research Institutes, Inc. (formerly Narcotic and Drug Research, Inc.) and its subcontractor, the Association for Drug Abuse Prevention and Treatment (ADAPT), in the Williamsburg section of Brooklyn from February 1988 to September 1990.

The project aimed to *organise* IDUs against AIDS and to *mobilise* their peer influence in enhancing the culture of risk reduction. One of the objectives of this project was to develop a drug users' organisation, similar to the ones mentioned earlier in this chapter. In practice, it was *organising from the outside*, with the effort initiated and run by an ex-user project staff rather than by active IDUs; details of this are discussed elsewhere (Friedman et al., 1992). The methods applied in this community-level intervention included intensive street outreach, leader identification and development, organising collective events (such as the clean-up of an abandoned building where a number of drug injectors lived and where shooting galleries were located); conducting weekly group meetings and health fairs; providing one-on-one counselling and referral services; and distributing risk reduction materials (including condoms, bleach kits and educational pamphlets). The project also occasionally published a newsletter which covered topics related to AIDS and health care, and carried announcements of weekly group meetings, community events and other information relevant to the community. For local IDUs, the project storefront served as a 'hang-out' and 'drop-in' centre and a place to seek assistance in medical and social service emergencies. The underlying focus of these efforts was to convince IDUs that they should reduce their risks and to develop a mutually reinforced subculture of risk-free behaviours among them.

The project was of limited duration. It was part of a larger project that was funded for three years. Disagreements between the parties to the project about whether it should focus on organising drug users or whether the bulk of its activities should be concentrated on providing individual counselling and assistance (supplemented by some educational outreach in which bleach and condoms would be distributed) meant that it was impossible to seek continued funding, and also that no lasting drug users' organisation was established. Efforts to establish a permanent leadership were hindered by the reluctance of some organising staff to see drug users as capable of being leaders (particularly on the part of staff who believed in the tenets of Narcotics Anonymous or of therapeutic communities that see drug use *per se* as leading to incompetence). More generally, staff tended to get advice from the drug injectors who were part of meetings, but maintained the right to make their own decisions and to organise on their own terms – all of which are exactly what the community organising literature cautions against doing since this prevents the development of self-confidence among the people being organised and keeps them from 'taking ownership' of the project and thus becoming deeply committed to it (Burghardt, 1982; Kahn, 1970).

In spite of all these difficulties, the data provided below indicate that interventions which attempt to use mobilisation and subcultural change to produce behavioural change can be successful in leading to risk reduction.

BEHAVIOURAL OUTCOMES OF OUTSIDE ORGANISING

The organising intervention aimed to encourage HIV risk reduction in two ways: by a direct individual-level effect among IDUs (and their sexual partners) who were personally in contact with the project; and by an indirect or community-level effect through diffusion of behavioural changes from those in direct contact with the project to the larger IDU community through changes in subcultural norms.

While the service aspect of the project was under way in Williamsburg, we studied behavioural changes by interviewing IDUs in the neighbourhood. The baseline interviews were done using the NIDA AIDS Initial Assessment (AIA) questionnaire. Subjects who answered the baseline questionnaire were followed up and re-interviewed after about six months using the AIDS Follow-up Assessment (AFA) questionnaire. These questionnaires covered information on background characteristics, health status, social contacts, involvement in activities organised by the project, drug use behaviours, and detailed information on sexual activity. Of the 628 eligible IDUs interviewed at intake, 397 (63 per cent) were followed up. The mean average follow-up interval was 7.3 months.

As shown in Table 14.1, changes occurred in a wide range of risk behaviours among IDUs in the neighbourhood. These are indicative of the positive effects of community organisation and related peer mobilisation efforts. In addition, 46 per cent of the sample reported at follow-up that they

Table 14.1 Community-level changes in drug use risk behaviours

Risk behaviour	Intake		Follow-up		Change*
	N	Freq/%	N	Freq/%	
Drug injection frequency	628	172	397	114	−58
Shooting gallery use	625	23	350	15	−8
Renting used syringes	611	7	350	4	−3
Lending used syringes	611	11	349	8	−3
Sharing cookers or cotton	611	33	350	28	−5
Sharing rinse water	611	28	350	20	−8
Using wrapped syringes only once	611	22	350	36	14
Using new syringes	626	59	348	72	13
Cleaning syringes with bleach	550	28	287	45	17
Injecting at own place	625	28	350	48	20

*$p<0.05$

had entered drug abuse treatment since their intake interview. More than 59 per cent also reported that they had taught someone about cleaning used syringes with bleach, indicating that the project activities helped mobilise IDUs to initiate and spread bleach use information among other IDUs in the community.

Focusing in particular on sexual risk reduction changes (i.e. increased condom use) among IDUs in the neighbourhood, three measures of condom use are employed both for the six months prior to intake interview and for the period between the intake and follow-up. These are: the proportion of IDUs who reported ever using a condom, the proportion who reported always using condoms, and the proportion of sexual acts in which a condom was used.

As Figure 14.1 shows, all three measures show condom use to have increased among IDUs between intake and follow-up. The percentage of IDUs ever using a condom increased from 53 per cent at intake to 61 per cent ($p<0.03$) at follow-up. Those who always used condoms increased from 26 per cent to 34 per cent ($p<0.02$), and the mean percentage of sexual encounters in which a condom was used increased from 40 per cent to 48 per cent ($p<0.008$). Ethnographic data also show supporting evidence of aggregate-level behavioural changes in condom use among the IDU community in the neighbourhood.

Further analyses of consistent condom use are limited to a sample of 282 individuals who were followed up and had sex at both intake and follow-up. It should be mentioned that the levels of condom use at intake among subjects who were followed up did not differ significantly from those of subjects who were not followed up (25 per cent vs 27 per cent; $p<0.67$). Among those who were followed up, condom use (at follow-up) did not vary significantly by

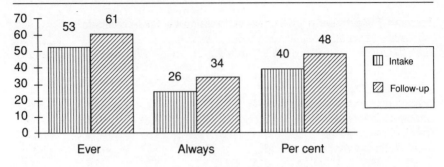

Figure 14.1 Overall condom use levels among IDUs in Williamsburg at intake and follow-up

gender, race/ethnicity, religion or by duration of drug injection experience. A significantly higher proportion of IDUs who engaged in commercial sex work always used condoms at follow-up. We did not have data to examine whether levels of condom use varied by subjects' HIV status or by partners' drug injection status.

As part of the organising intervention, the project arranged group meetings for men, for women and for HIV-positive injectors. These sessions encouraged mutual peer support, and covered topics related to HIV transmission, antibody testing, drug treatment, safer injection and safer sex, along with other topics of general concern to the group. The attendance of subjects at any of these meetings was considered as a measure of direct programme participation. Condom use levels at follow-up were consistently higher for direct programme participants than for non-participants. Almost half (49 per cent) of those who ever attended a project group meeting always used condoms at follow-up, whereas only 29 per cent of non-participants did so (p<0.001). This relationship remains true within the subset of IDUs who engaged in commercial sex work.

There was a significant increase in consistent condom use between intake and follow-up among IDUs who attended group meetings. Although of a lesser magnitude, the proportion always using condoms also increased among IDUs who never attended a project group meeting. This may imply a possible secular trend in condom use which may also be indicative of an indirect community-level effect of the organising project efforts among IDUs in the neighbourhood.

A multivariate analysis was carried out to determine the independent predictors of always using condoms during the follow-up period (with condom use at intake forced into the model as a control variable so the equation would measure the predictors of change in condom use). Independent variables with univariate p<0.10 were included in a stepwise logistic regression equation (forward selection and backward elimination). The goodness-of-fit of the model was tested with the Hosmer–Lemeshow statistic (Hosmer and Lemeshow, 1989).

Table 14.2 Predictors of consistent condom use at follow-up (Stepwise logistic regression results)

Independent variables	Odds ratio	95% C.I	p
Always using condoms at intake	8.77	4.08–18.8	0.001
Engaging in commercial sex work	2.04	0.99–4.23	0.056
Changing from multiple to single partner	0.30	0.01–0.90	0.033
Age 35 or above	2.12	1.03–4.34	0.040
Attending project group meeting	2.46	1.18–5.13	0.017

Model Chi-square = 61.4 with 5 DF (p = 0.0001)
Hosmer-Lemeshow goodness-of-fit statistic = 5.6 with 8 DF (p = 0.6873)

Final multivariate logistic results are presented in Table 14.2. From the coefficient on intake condom use status (odds ratio 8.8), it is evident that there was a strong tendency among IDUs in Williamsburg toward maintenance of consistent condom use. Those who changed from multiple-partner sex at intake to single-partner sex at follow-up were less likely always to use condoms at follow-up than others. Direct programme participation as measured by meeting attendance remained significant as an independent predictor of consistent condom use at follow-up. Engaging in commercial sex work also tended to be a determinant of consistent condom use at the multivariate level (p<0.057). Nearly 38 per cent of those who engaged in commercial sex work were consistent condom users at intake itself. This is probably because many commercial sex workers attended the project's women's groups prior to baseline interviews taking place and many of these groups were particularly active in the initial stages of the intervention.

One result to be mentioned is relapse from consistent condom use by IDUs. Among those who were consistent condom users at intake, 29 per cent failed to maintain consistent condom use during the follow-up period. Nearly two-thirds (63 per cent) of subjects in this group had multiple sex partners at intake, whereas at follow-up half of them engaged in sex only with one partner – an organising project message somewhat followed by the community.

METHODOLOGICAL LIMITATIONS

Certain methodological constraints limited our ability to study individual and community-level changes, and thus also, the effectiveness of the organising intervention. One of these was loss of subjects to follow up. This was in part a result of the project having targeted a neighbourhood with a particularly destitute and homeless group of IDUs (follow-up was made difficult because of a lack of fixed addresses), in part because gentrification became widespread in the neighbourhood during the course of the project (which drove many subjects out of the neighbourhood), and in part because out-of-treatment IDUs are a particularly difficult population to follow up.

Second, among those who were followed up, more than one-third (36 per cent) exhibited a change in the number of sex partners between intake and follow-up. Of the total sample, 98 IDUs (25 per cent) did not have sex during the six months prior to intake; 32 per cent of this group became sexually active during the follow-up period. Among the 289 subjects who were sexually active in the six months prior to intake, 46 (16 per cent) did not engage in sex during the follow-up period. These shifts between categories created analytical problems when studying individual-level changes in condom use. In particular, since the analysis of individual-level change in condom use was limited to those who had sex during both intake and follow-up periods, the number of subjects in these analyses was considerably decreased.

A third issue was the differences in the timing of initiation of the intervention and the timing of the survey, which imposed another limit on evaluating the effectiveness of the intervention. The organising efforts were already under way prior to subjects' initial interviews, so by baseline some subjects would have been influenced by both the direct and the indirect effects mentioned earlier. Thus, the difference between baseline and follow-up provides only a conservative estimate of change.

Fourth, the non-experimental before-and-after design used in the analysis limits the confidence of conclusions that the intervention was the cause of the observed risk reduction. Secular trends and/or the influence of other ongoing intervention programmes in New York City may also have caused them. However, given the expense and logistical difficulties in evaluating community-level interventions, an experimental design was considered unfeasible.

CONCLUSIONS

IDUs have set up and run drug users' organisations on at least three continents. These organisations have made important contributions to local and national HIV and drug policy, have provided risk reduction services such as outreach and syringe exchange, as well as succour for the ill, and have been able to conceive and implement long-term strategies for HIV prevention and for organisational growth. In all cases, they have accomplished this in the face of considerable scepticism among drug abuse treatment agencies, public health officials, and the general public. Of course, drug users' groups have had their organisational ups, downs, and at times complete collapses – as do all forms of voluntary organisations, corporations, and indeed whole industries. Nevertheless, the overall performance of drug users' organisations has been far more impressive than could have been conceived of by proponents of the conventional wisdom that drug users are personally too disorganised by their addictions and pre-existing mental disorders. Indeed, we would argue that the extent to which drug users' organisations have been able to establish themselves and undertake risk reduction throws into doubt those theories of drug addiction which view heavy drug use as inevitably leading to incompetence.

Nonetheless, we should also consider the limitations of drug users' organisations as actors in the fight against AIDS. Like all community organisations, they sometimes undergo periods of infighting and organisational rupture. Furthermore, they are functioning in a social environment that is often chaotic – and may become more so due to police or other pressures – and often with groups characterised by unmet economic and medical needs. Thus, the impact of drug user organisations may at times be restricted, even if their actions suffice to sustain safer injection norms in a local IDU community. Where the pressures of law enforcement and social stigmatisation lead groups of drug injectors underground, this may limit the extent of an organisation's normative and behavioural influence.

Little formal research has yet been done on drug users' organisations – whether about their organisational development or about their behavioural impacts so as yet it is impossible to provide definitive answers to whether they have 'worked' as an HIV prevention strategy. The fact that HIV transmission rates among IDUs are very low in Australia – where drug users' organisations are an integral part of AIDS prevention strategy – is suggestive, but is by no means proof of effectiveness. There is an increasing need for descriptive as well as formal research on drug user groups and their efficacy in preventing drug-related health damage and in promoting safe, healthier behaviour among IDUs.

The results of the outside organising effort among IDUs in New York are also encouraging, even though internal considerations and funding limitations meant that no lasting organisation of IDUs was formed. There were considerable decreases in risk behaviour. The increase in condom use was particularly notable. Sexual behavioural changes have clearly lagged behind drug use behavioural changes. Condom use is still sporadic among a large number of IDUs in many communities. Our data indicate that organising peer support and promulgating ideas that drug injectors (and their sexual partners) should work together to protect each other against HIV could contribute towards overcoming some of the barriers to condom use and to initiating modifications in sexual behaviour.

We need to develop ways to ensure that risk reducing behavioural changes remain stable or increase over time. To the extent that safer sex and safer injection practices become normatively sanctioned (where violators of norms face dissuasion, ostracism or worse), behavioural changes should be more stable. The existence of drug users organisations fighting to maintain and strengthen such norms from within the subculture should help to do this. The organising approach to risk elimination should be developed, implemented and tested on a wider scale.

Finally, this chapter shows that even drug injectors can organise against

AIDS, despite the difficulties created by addiction, police pressure and social ostracism. This points to the fact that other groups faced with threats to their health can also organise for behavioural change and for changes in social policies and institutions that contribute to their health problems. Worldwide experience indicates that such efforts can help reduce occupational health risks and can reduce local levels of environmental pollution, as well as helping to prevent the spread of infectious diseases such as HIV. Beyond this, such efforts can sometimes contribute to wider social changes, such as when environmental movements in Eastern Europe helped produce the transformation of 1989.

REFERENCES

Abdul-Quader, A. S., Tross, S., Friedman, S. R., Kouzi, A. C. and Des Jarlais, D. C. (1990) 'Street-recruited intravenous drug users and sexual risk reduction in New York City', *AIDS*, 4: 1075–1079.

Abdul-Quader, A.S., Des Jarlais D. C., Tross, S., McCoy, E., Morales, G. and Velez, I. (1992) 'Outreach to injecting drug users and female sexual partners of drug users on the Lower East Side of New York', *British Journal of Addiction*, 87: 681–688.

Adam, B. (1987) *The Rise of a Gay and Lesbian Movement*, Boston: Twayne.

Altman, D. (1991) 'The primacy of politics: organising around AIDS', *AIDS*, 5 (suppl. 2): S231–S238.

Becker, M. H. and Joseph J.G. (1988) 'AIDS and behavioral change to reduce risk: A review', *American Journal of Public Health* 78: 394–410.

Broadhead, R.S. (1991) 'Social constructions of bleach in combating AIDS among injection drug users', *Journal of Drug Issues,* 21: 711–734.

Broadhead, R. S. and Fox, K. J. (1990) 'Takin' it to the streets: AIDS outreach as ethnography', *Journal of Contemporary Ethnography*, 19: 322–348.

Burghardt, S. (1982) *The Other Side of Organising*, Cambridge, MA: Schenkman.

Burrows, D. and Price, C. (1993) 'Peer education among IDUs in Baltimore and Sydney: similarities and differences within a model of peer education'. Paper presented at IX International Conference on AIDS, Berlin [session WS–D09–6].

CDC (Centers for Disease Control) (1991) 'Drug use and sexual behaviours among sex partners of injecting drug users – United States, 1988–1990', *Morbidity and Mortality Weekly Report*, 40: 855–860.

Coutinho, R., van Grievson, G. and Moss, A. (1989) 'Effects of preventive efforts among homosexual men', *AIDS*, 3 (suppl. 1): S53–S56.

Des Jarlais, D. C. and Friedman, S. R. (1992a) 'AIDS prevention programmes for intravenous drug users', in G. P. Wormser (ed.) *AIDS and other Manifestations of HIV Infection. Second Edition* (pp. 645–658), New York: Raven Press.

Des Jarlais, D. C. and Friedman, S. R. (1992b) 'The AIDS epidemic and legal access to sterile equipment for injecting illicit drugs', *Annals of the American Academy of Political and Social Science*, 521: 42–65.

Des Jarlais, D. C., Abdul-Quader, A. and Tross, S. (1991) 'The next problem: maintenance of AIDS risk reduction among injecting drug users', *International Journal of Addiction*, 26: 1279–1292.

Des Jarlais, D. C., Friedman, S. R., Choopanya, K., Vanichseni, S. and Ward, T. P. (1992) 'International epidemiology of HIV and AIDS among injecting drug users', *AIDS*, 6: 1053–1068.

Dolan K. A., Stimson, G. V. and Donoghoe, M. C. (1993) 'Reductions in HIV risk behaviours and stable HIV prevalence in syringe-exchange clients and other injectors in England', *Drug and Alcohol Review*, 12: 133–142.

Friedman, S. R. (1993) 'Going beyond education to mobilizing subcultural change', in National Committee on AIDS Control and National Institute on Alcohol and Drugs, *Encouraging Peer Support for Risk Reduction among Injecting Drug Users*, Amsterdam.

Friedman, S. R., Des Jarlais, D. C., Sotheran, J. L., et al. (1987) 'AIDS and self-organization among intravenous drug users', *International Journal of Addiction*, 22: 201–219.

Friedman, S. R., de Jong, W. M. and Des Jarlais, D. C. (1988) 'Problems and dynamics of organising intravenous drug users for AIDS prevention', *Health Education Research*, 3: 49–57.

Friedman, S. R., Sufian, M., Curtis, R., Neaigus, A. and Des Jarlais, D. C. (1992) 'Organising drug users against AIDS', in J. Huber and B. E. Schneider (eds) *The Social Context of AIDS* (pp. 115–130), Newbury, CA: Sage.

Friedman, S. R., de Jong, W. and Wodak, A. (1993a) 'Community development as a response to HIV among drug injectors', *AIDS*, 7 (suppl. 1): S263–S269.

Friedman, S. R., Jose B., Neaigus A., et al. (1993b) 'Widespread condom use by seropositive injecting drug users with non-injector sexual partners', paper presented at IX International Conference on AIDS, Berlin [session PO–C11–2847].

Friedman, S. R., Rodriguez-Arenas, A., Zunzunegui-Pastro, V., Wenston, J., Sotheran, J. L. and Des Jarlais D. C. (1993c) 'Similarities in syringe-sharing among drug injectors in Madrid and New York City', paper presented at 121 Annual Meeting of the American Public Health Association, San Francisco, October [session 3250].

Friedman S.R., Des Jarlais D.C. and Ward T.P. (1994) 'Social models for changing risk behaviour', in J. Peterson and R. DiClemente (eds) *Preventing AIDS: Theory and Practice of Behavioural Interventions*, New York: Plenum.

Grund, J. P. C. (1993) 'Drug use as a social ritual: functionality, symbolism and determinants of self-regulation', Doctoral Dissertation, Rotterdam: Erasmus University.

Hartgers, C., Buning, E. C., van Santen, G. W. et al. (1989) 'The impact of the needle and syringe exchange programme in Amsterdam on injecting risk behaviour', *AIDS*, 3: 571–576.

Hosmer, D. W, and Lemeshow, S. (1989) *Applied Logistic Regression*, New York: John Wiley.

Jain, S., Flynn, N., Bailey, V. et al. (1989) 'IVDU and AIDS: more resistance to changing their sexual than their needle-sharing practices', paper presented at V International Conference on AIDS, Montreal [abstract WDP79].

Jose, B., Friedman, S.R., Neaigus, A. et al. (1993) 'Syringe-mediated drug-sharing (backloading): a new risk factor for HIV among injecting drug users', *AIDS*, 7: 1653–1660.

Kahn, S. (1970) *How People Get Power*, New York: McGraw-Hill.

Kayal, P. M. (1993) *Bearing Witness: Gay Men's Health Crisis and the Politics of AIDS*, Boulder, CO: Westview Press.

Kelly, J. A., St Lawrence, J. S., Diaz, Y. E., Stevenson, L. Y., Hauth, A. C., Brasfeld, T. L., Kalichman, S. C., Smith, J. E. and Andrew, M. E. (1991) 'HIV risk behavior reduction following intervention with key opinion leaders of population: an experimental analysis', *American Journal of Public Health*, 81: 168–171.

Kelly, J. A., St Lawrence, J. S., Stevenson, L. Y., Hauth, A. C., Kalichman, S. C., Diaz, Y. E., Brasfeld, T. L., Koob, J. J. and Morgan, M. G. (1992) 'Community AIDS/HIV risk reduction: the effects of endorsements by popular people in three cities' *American Journal of Public Health*, 82: 1483–1489.

McAlister, A., Puska, P., Salonen, J. T., Tuomilehto, J. and Koskela, K. (1982)

'Theory and action for health promotion: illustrations from the North Karelia Project', *American Journal of Public Health*, 72: 43–50.

McKeganey, N. and Barnard, M. (1992) *AIDS, Drugs and Sexual Risk: Lives in the Balance*, Buckingham, Open University Press.

Marmor, M., Des Jarlais, D. C., Cohen, H. *et al.* (1987) 'Risk factors and infection with human immunodeficiency virus among intravenous drug abusers in New York City' *AIDS*, 1: 39–44.

Morales, E. S. and Fullilove, M.T. (1992) '"Many are called . . .": participation by minority leaders in an AIDS intervention in San Francisco', *Ethnicity and Disease*, 2: 389–401.

Neaigus, A., Sufian, M., Friedman, S. R. *et al.* (1990a) 'Effects of outreach intervention on risk reduction among intravenous drug users', *AIDS Education and Prevention*, 2: 253–271.

Neaigus, A., Friedman, S. R., Sufian, M., Stepherson, B., Goldsmith, D. S. and Mota, P. (1990b) 'Effects of peer culture, race, and gender on IV drug use risk reduction'. Paper presented at 118th Annual Meeting of the American Public Health Association, New York City, October.

Neaigus, A., Friedman, S. R., Jose, B., *et al.* (1993) 'Syringe-sharing and social characteristics of drug-injecting dyads', paper presented at 121st Annual Meeting of the American Public Health Association, San Francisco, October [session 3137].

Newmeyer, J. A. (1988) 'Why bleach? Development of a strategy to combat HIV contagion among San Francisco intravenous drug users', in R. J. Battjes and R. W. Pickens (eds) *Needle Sharing among Intravenous Drug Users: National and International Perspectives* (pp. 151–159). Washington, DC: US Government Printing Office, NIDA Research Monograph 80.

Newmeyer, J. A., Feldman, H. W., Biernacki, P. and Watters, J. K. (1989) 'Preventing AIDS contagion among intravenous drug users', *Medical Anthropology,* 10: 167–175.

Ogburn, W. F. (1922) *Social Change*, New York: Huebsch.

Puska, P., Nissinen, A., Tuomilehto, J., Salonen, J.Y., Koskela, K., McAlister, A., Kottke, T. E., Macoby, N. and Farquhar, J. W. (1985) 'The community-based strategy to prevent coronary heart disease: conclusions from ten years of the North Karelia project', *Annual Review of Public Health*, 6: 147–193.

Quimby, E., and Friedman, S. R. (1989) 'Dynamics of Black mobilisation against AIDS in New York City', *Social Problems*, 36: 403–415.

Rogers, E. M. (1982) *Diffusion of Innovations. Third Edition*, New York: Free Press.

Rogers, E. M. and Shoemaker, F. F. (1971) *Communication of Innovation: A Cross-cultural Approach, Second Edition*, New York: Free Press.

Schoenbaum, E.E, Hartel, D., Selwyn, P.A. *et al.* (1989) 'Risk factors for HIV-1 infection in intravenous drug abusers', *New England Journal of Medicine*, 321: 874–879.

Sibthorpe B. (1992) 'The social construction of sexual relationships as a determinant of HIV risk perception and condom use among injection drug users', *Medical Anthropology Quarterly*, 6: 255–270.

Sotheran, J. L. (1991) 'HIV risk and social relationships among IV drug users', paper presented at Annual Workshop on Psychosocial Factors in Population Change, Washington, DC, 19–20 March.

Stall, R., Coates, T. and Hoff, C. (1988) 'Behavioral risk reduction for HIV infection among gay and bisexual men', *American Psychologist*, 43: 878–885.

Tilly, C. (1978) *From Mobilisation to Revolution*, Reading, MA: Addison-Wesley.

Tross, S., Abdul-Quader, A., Silvert, H. *et al.* (1992) 'Condom use among male injecting drug users, New York City, 1987–1990', *Morbidity and Mortality Weekly Report*, 41: 617–619

Watkins, K.E., Metzger, D., Woody, G. and McLellan, A.T. (1993) 'Determinants of condom use among intravenous drug users', *AIDS*, 7: 719–723.

Watters, J. K., Cheng, Y., Segal, M., Lorvick, J., Case, P. and Carlson, J. (1990) 'Epidemiology and prevention of HIV in intravenous drug users in San Francisco, 1986–1989', paper presented at Sixth International Conference on AIDS, San Francisco, CA [abstract FC106].

Wiebel, W. (1988) 'Combining ethnographic and epidemiologic methods for targeted AIDS interventions: the Chicago model', in R. J. Battjes and R. W. Pickens (eds) *Needle Sharing among Intravenous Drug Abusers: National and International Perspectives*, Washington, DC: US Government Printing Office, NIDA Research Monograph 80.

Wiebel, W., Fritz, R. and Chene, D. (1989) 'Description of intervention procedures utilized by the AIDS Outreach Intervention Projects – University of Illinois at Chicago, School of Public Health', in *Proceedings of the Community Epidemiology Work Group: Chicago – June 1989* (vol. III, pp. 68–79), Rockville, MD: National Institute on Drug Abuse.

Index